Communicating Across Dementia

Stephen Miller

A How To Book

ROBINSON

First published in Great Britain in 2015 by Robinson

1 3 5 7 9 10 8 6 4 2

Important note:
This book is not intended as a substitute for medical advice or treatment. Any person with a condition requiring medical attention should consult a qualified medical practitioner or suitable therapist.

A CIP catalogue record for this book
is available from the British Library.

ISBN 978-1-84528-570-8 (paperback)
ISBN 978-1-47211-478-5 (ebook)

Typeset in Times New Roman by TW Typesetting, Plymouth, Devon
Printed and bound in Great Britain by CPI Mackays

Robinson
is an imprint of
Constable & Robinson Ltd
100 Victoria Embankment
London EC4Y 0DY

An Hachette UK Company
www.hachette.co.uk

www.constablerobinson.com

How To Books are published by Constable & Robinson, a part of Little Brown Book Group. We welcome proposals from authors who have first-hand experience of their subjects. Please set out the aims of your book, its target market and its suggested contents in an email to Nikki.Read@howtobooks.co.uk.

For Pat – you taught me a lot.

'Such a precious thing, a thought expressed.'

Sally Magnusson (from *Where Memories Go*)

Contents

1

Introduction

When a person is told that they have, or probably have, dementia they are at the start of a journey. However, it is not a journey they will make alone; you will be there, too – at least for some of the time. The condition has a major impact on everyday life, which increases as the years go by, and a person with dementia needs your help and support.

Who are you, by the way? Well, you might be a wife, a husband, a daughter, a son, a grandchild, some other relative, or perhaps a close friend; you might live with the person or near them, visit regularly or occasionally.

Alternatively, you might be someone with an interest in a very topical subject that will almost certainly affect someone you know.

The focus of this book is communication and the human interaction that is an essential element of that communication. Together they constitute a lifeline for people with dementia, a lifeline that has the potential to enable their voices to be heard – their concerns, wishes, opinions and memories. Dementia in its various forms changes and diminishes a person's ability to communicate over time; and the longer that person lives, the greater the degree of diminution.

The principal aim of this book is to demonstrate that there are numerous ways in which a person's communicative capabilities and experiences can be maintained and enhanced for a considerable length of time. This in turn has the potential to reduce the stress often experienced by people with dementia and those who care for them. Dementia affects people's lives in many ways, but one thing is certain – the better the quality of communication that can be achieved, the better the quality of life that can be maintained.

And I mean receptive and expressive communication in the very broadest sense, not just conversation – though that is of course very important. Everything a person experiences via each of their senses, for example:

◆ Looking at photographs, people-watching.
◆ Reading signs or newspapers.
◆ Watching films.
◆ Listening to music or birdsong.
◆ Choosing clothes.
◆ Stroking a cat, kneading dough.
◆ Enjoying aromas.
◆ Eating a favourite food from childhood.
◆ Making love.
◆ Considering the terms of a will.

The only limit is your imagination.

In addition, there is the vast world of non-verbal communication – you can say a great deal with a friendly smile, a thumbs-up sign or an arm around the shoulder. There are also lots of ways to communicate information to people with a variety of aids: calendars, explanatory signs or time-appropriate lighting discreetly deployed around the house.

When you start to look at things in this way, you soon see that there are lots of practical and effective opportunities for enhancing communication. A person with dementia wants to be able to benefit from these things – but they need your help – increasingly so, as time goes by.

It is always important to accentuate the positive. Too often you hear people talking about what a person with dementia cannot *do as a result of their condition; your challenge is to find and exploit the things they* can *do.*

There has been a great deal of coverage of dementia in the media in recent years. The number of people who have the condition is substantial and is growing. This can probably be attributed to greater awareness of the condition, earlier diagnosis and the simple fact that people are living longer than in the past. When a person is given a diagnosis, or probable diagnosis, the chances are that they have already been living with the condition for some time. Relatives often look back and remember incidents which seemed strange or out of character and then realize that was probably the start.

Within a few years there are likely to be more than a million people with some type of dementia in the UK. The most common is Alzheimer's disease, which accounts for roughly 60 per cent of cases. After that comes vascular dementia (associated with problems of supply of blood to the brain) at around 20 per cent. There are other less common types as well. More details of the types of dementia and their particular symptoms and features can be found on the websites of organizations such as the Alzheimer's Society. The condition is more likely to begin in later life, although a significant minority of cases develop earlier, when people are in their fifties or early sixties.

DEMENTIA IN THE PAST

Until comparatively recently there was a great deal of negative comment associated with dementia. People might say that the person had died but the body lived on. People working in care homes might say dismissively, 'You won't get much out of him', or compare people with dementia walking around the home to goldfish in a glass bowl. This kind of thinking has resulted in a great many people with dementia simply having their physical needs attended to while their feelings of isolation or loneliness and their desire for stimulation have largely been ignored. The widespread use of phrases like 'dementia victim' is also negative since it risks defining people in terms of their condition – an old person, helpless and hopeless. The countless events that went into making up the person's life are easily lost from view with attitudes like this.

Would you ever like to be regarded in this way?

Although I didn't realize it at the time, I came across dementia early on in my life. I took a summer job at a hospital in Glasgow when I left school in 1970. It had been arranged through a friend who said it would probably involve ferrying patients around and cleaning floors. In fact I worked as a nursing assistant and was involved in many aspects of personal care for a wide variety of patients – something that would be unthinkable nowadays.

The hospital was a throwback to Victorian times. I was told it was a 'dustbin' where patients were 'dumped' when there was nothing more that could be done for them. I am sure that many of them had some form of dementia. It was a depressing place, but looking back what strikes me above all was that there was no attempt to provide any kind of stimulation whatsoever for the patients. They were simply helped out of bed in the morning, dressed, washed, put in chairs and then left to spend most of the day staring into space. The major events of the day were the tea trolley, mealtimes and drugs rounds. It seems incredible, looking back, that the authorities thought it was acceptable to treat people in this way.

Visiting time was the worst. Relatives and friends rarely came and so the staff took it on themselves to sit and chat to the patients for a few minutes, just to give them some kind of companionable experience. I suspect that if someone had suggested the patients should have been respected as people, and that ways should have been found to provide stimulation and improve communication with them, the authorities of the day would have been completely mystified.

Apart from an efficient electrical system and reliable hot and cold running water, I doubt if the place was any different from the Frankfurt asylum in which Doctor Alois Alzheimer treated his patients at the start of the twentieth century.

HOW THINGS HAVE MOVED ON

A great deal has changed for the better. There is far greater openness about the condition, thanks in part to the publicity given to high-profile people such as Terry Pratchett, Ronald Reagan, Iris Murdoch, Rita Hayworth and Prunella Scales; this has also helped to reduce stigma. Much more attention is paid to the psychological and emotional needs of people with dementia, and their right to high standards of care has been enshrined in various statutes and government initiatives throughout the UK.

One of the most important advances has been to treat people with dementia as human beings who are to be respected, not merely problems to be managed – and to enable them to remain active participants in the world for as long as possible.

Better communication makes such goals more achievable.

There are brilliant scientific researchers working on earlier diagnosis, more effective drugs and possible cures. What they do is very impressive, but major breakthroughs in these fields are for the future – and this book is not about any of that.

It is about the here and now and making all aspects of communication as good as possible with a view to making life better for people with dementia – and those looking after them face-to-face, on a day-to-day basis. There are many experts in a variety of fields working hard to achieve these goals at the present time.

CONSIDERING YOUR ROLE

If you find yourself in a situation where someone very close to you, in particular a spouse or one of your parents, has been given a diagnosis or a probable diagnosis of some form of dementia, I would like to encourage you to reflect on your role – a role that has been thrust upon you by events. Some people who write about looking after people with dementia seem to make certain assumptions. Two important ones go something like this:

1. You always loved and got on really well with the person.

2. Now that the person has dementia, you have large amounts of free time available to think of ways to make their life better.

Sometimes this is true – indeed you might see the care of a relative with dementia as your main mission in life. I remember one lady I met several years ago who did just that. Her husband had a particularly aggressive form of dementia. She said he had always been a good husband and now it was 'payback time'. In reality, however, a close relative, let alone a friend, will find it very difficult to devote themselves to a person with dementia to anything like this extent – and they should not feel guilty about it.

You might be at an age when you have a lot of responsibilities in life, concerns over money or your children or your job, or perhaps your own or your partner's health. You might find yourself in a situation where you are one of three children but one emigrated years ago and the other lives in another part of the country, so most of the load falls on you. The realization that you are the one who will be expected to do the lion's share of the work might strike you as unfair. Perhaps you did not have a very close relationship with the person. Maybe you never even particularly liked them.

Feelings of resentment are hard to avoid in such real-life situations.

Perhaps none of these things applies in your case – if so, you are almost certainly in the minority. Whatever the circumstances, here are some points I think you should consider as you mull over the hand of cards you have been dealt:

The person with dementia has been an important figure in your life – and now has a life-diminishing condition and needs your help. You have it within your power to make their life better.

The chances are you are not prepared for the challenges of looking after a person with dementia. But how could you be? The person is someone with whom you have enjoyed what might be termed a normal relationship, with little or no element of caring. You have done things together, gone to the cinema, enjoyed family occasions, shared jokes, tears and had some disagreements. Nobody is really prepared, unless they happen to be health professionals working in the field; but this is true of many other conditions, from cancer to motor neurone disease.

Now everything has changed. It is hard. You are on the spot, but remember you are not the only one; many others are faced with similar life situations.

The person is still the same person you have known for so many years. Older people often say that inside they feel exactly the same as they did when they were twenty-one. Don't you? It's the same with people with dementia – it's just that the person you know so well can now be harder to see, much harder as time passes. The difficulties caused by dementia go well beyond normal ageing and so substantial adaptations have to be made

in order to make life better for them – but you must try not to
lose sight of the fact that the person is still there. It's a major
challenge.

*I think you should try to accept this and give the person as much
of your time as you can reasonably spare. You really can make a
positive difference.*

Considerable benefits you might not have thought about

**By spending time with the person you will have the
opportunity to get to know them better.** It might be that you
have some guilt feelings from the past – if the person is a parent,
did you give them a hard time when you were a teenager? Did
you forget birthdays? Did you fail to appreciate the challenges
they faced when they were younger and when you were growing
up? Perhaps you will start to understand the world more from
their point of view and make sense of difficulties or resentments
you might have felt in the past. I believe that deep down
everybody wants to get on well with their parents. The kind of
close and intimate contact involved in looking after a person
with dementia presents opportunities for revisiting the past in
positive ways.

**If the person is one of your parents, they knew you from the
start.** They know things about you and your early life that you
are unaware of. As part of the process of being with them, you
might discover snatches of information about yourself that you
were previously unaware of. It is true that memory is damaged
by dementia, but the things the person will remember best are
the things from long ago. By helping them to express themselves

you might well be able to do a bit of personal historical research. As the condition progresses, parts of you will be lost beyond recall. This is life; all the more reason to be closely involved with the person at this time.

You will come into contact with other relatives or family friends you have not seen for a long time. As part of the process of being involved in the care of a close relative or friend, this is very likely. It could result in the strengthening of old bonds and the creation of new ones.

Finding ways to enhance communication can be an extremely rewarding activity. You look at a situation that is problematic, work out a plan to make it better, apply it, and have the satisfaction of seeing it make a difference in practice. By coming up with ways to improve a person's ability to communicate, whether to find out what is bothering them or what kind of activity pleases them, or simply to express their thoughts more clearly, you will be making the care management of the person easier and help to reduce stress levels all round.

You will acquire an important skill. There is a great demand for help and assistance for the care of people with dementia and you could open up the possibility of rewarding work, paid or voluntary, if you develop a knack for improving the quality of life of a person with dementia.

Your thoughts and advice will be greatly valued – once you have gained experience. Given the increase in the prevalence of dementia you will doubtless come across friends who are also faced with the challenges of caring for a person with dementia.

There is a widespread view – to which I subscribe – that the longer a person can remain in their own home, the more contentment and security they will experience as their condition progresses. It follows that anything which can be done to make management of the situation easier and less stressful will help to achieve this goal. Even if every person with dementia only stayed at home for an extra year or two, that could add up to a significant benefit.

But although there are undoubtedly quite a number of positives, there is no getting away from the fact you will have to deal with some hardships.

Difficulties you will be faced with

◆ The very nature of the condition means that a person will become confused and forgetful, will probably ask the same questions and say the same things repeatedly, and will increasingly require a great deal of attention. With the best will in the world this can be extremely taxing.

◆ A person with dementia becomes less and less able to initiate things; they might appear flat and lacking enthusiasm. This can be exacerbated by medication. You might have the impression that they are not really bothered about doing the things they used to enjoy. This is often not true, but the onus is on you to make things happen. Sadly, even now, too many people with dementia are left for long spells without any meaningful activity or stimulation. How would you feel if it was you?

◆ As the condition progresses, you will be unable to share and discuss thoughts or feelings about it all with the person who has dementia, as you would if, say, they had cancer.

◆ Some of the people who have known the person in the past, friends or more distant relatives, might be less keen to maintain contact once the diagnosis becomes known. Previously, they might have had an easy-going, fun relationship with the person, which has now gone. They might feel uncomfortable and unsure about how to interact with the person. They might also be at an age and stage in life when they have their own health or family problems and these are their main priority. This is understandable and means that your role is even more important and valuable.

◆ There can be tensions and friction in the family, as decisions have to be taken about a wide range of care and financial issues.

◆ Above all, you will experience all the wretched sadness of watching a person, perhaps one of the most significant people in your life, appear to change inexorably before your eyes. It will seem at times that the person you knew so well is gradually sinking into a foggy quicksand which consumes large parts of who they are.

However, you will also find that with increased general awareness has come far greater understanding of the needs of those who care for people with dementia. As you approach the challenges of exploring the countless ways in which all forms of communication can be enhanced, try to see the process as a series of joint ventures. These will often involve just you and the person with dementia, but you should also get into the practice of enlisting the support of other people – willing friends and relatives, health professionals and so on. There are also numerous support groups for people with dementia and those who care for them. Spread the load.

Try to ensure also that you have time to yourself on a regular basis to pursue your own interests, or just relax. In this way you will be better equipped to help the person.

THE MOST IMPORTANT MESSAGES YOU NEED TO TAKE ON BOARD

When it comes to communication you must understand that *a person with dementia cannot change the way they are.*

Their conversation might be repetitive, they might not understand subtle jokes any more and they might not be able to follow plot lines of films as they did in the past; they also might not be able to chop vegetables in the easy and automatic way they used to, and they might behave rudely and inconsiderately at times. This may all be frustrating and disappointing but there is nothing they can do about it.

It follows therefore that *you are the one who has to change.*

Although you remain equals as fellow human beings, and family or other close relationships are theoretically unchanged, the reality is that as the condition becomes more advanced you will have to redefine your relationship. For many purposes your role will gradually change from that of an equal adult partner to, in addition, something like a special friend and facilitator. You must be prepared to adapt the way you interact with the person to make allowances for their condition. You have the power; the person with dementia is vulnerable and so it is incumbent on you to make changes but to do so considerately and responsibly in such a way that allows the person to maintain their dignity.

Following on from these basic points the next essential message on the subject of communication is: *The old ways will not work.*

To misquote a famous phrase: 'The past is a different country.' Perhaps you used to share sophisticated in-jokes, or had arguments about politics or football, or enjoyed visiting art galleries or playing cards or cooking meals together, or countless other things. There can be a temptation to try to continue to do the things you know the person used to like; you might well feel that in this way you are doing the best for them. This might work well in the early stages, but as the condition progresses it will gradually cease to be the case.

This can lead to frustration, irritation or even despondency. You might find yourself thinking, 'But he always used to like my jokes' or 'I remember she always loved that programme.' If you find yourself having these thoughts, red warning lights should come on. It is sad, but you have to come to terms with the fact that things have changed – and will gradually deteriorate further – and so you have change the way you do things.

This does not mean, however, that things are hopeless. Far from it. There are numerous ways in which communicative activities can and should be maintained. But you need to change, alter, recast, rejig, rethink, revisit (whatever word makes sense for you) the way you approach the whole subject of communication.

You should aim to acquire the skill – some would call it a knack – of assessing a situation that is not working or is problematic and then discreetly making changes or adaptations. This will mean the person is able to communicate more effectively and engage in activities that give pleasure for as long as possible.

It might be that a person always liked to watch police dramas on television. In the years following a diagnosis or probable diagnosis of dementia, they might well find these programmes difficult to follow and perhaps upsetting. However, you might assume that they will continue to get a lot out of them and that you are doing them a kindness by putting them on. This might well be a mistaken assumption. You need to be aware of the person's reactions – if it is clear that they become distracted and fidgety, don't follow the storyline and stop engaging with the programme then you have to take action.

The old way isn't working any more and to keep on trying the same thing over and over again runs the risk of upsetting the person not least because you will be reminding them of their failing powers.

It might be that you will find a nature programme on DVD, or perhaps an old home movie that the person can watch with enjoyment because there is not much mental processing involved.

This is not insulting or patronizing – merely a recognition of reality.

A person with dementia will gradually lose the ability to make adjustments in their life to suit their changing needs – which they would have done easily in the past. They need your help and one of your challenges will be to develop a mindset which looks out for the person, thinks for them at times, and seeks to initiate new ways of doing things – all without making the person feel useless or belittled.

This books aims to provide you with a wide range of strategies and ideas to help you become confident in making changes to the way you approach the whole subject of communication.

One other important point to bear in mind is this: Every person is different, but many people with dementia can lead near normal lives for a considerable length of time following diagnosis or probable diagnosis.

Many of the suggestions and strategies described in this book are aimed at people who have moved well beyond the early stages.

Even if you only take away a few important points or ideas that really work for you, reading this book will have been worthwhile. Going through the dementia journey with a person close to you can be hard at times, and nobody should pretend otherwise. However, it is equally true that, as with any life-diminishing condition, there are many ways to lessen the impact and ensure a good quality of life for many years.

2

The Key Role of Memory in Communication

At the heart of the difficulties caused by dementia is the way the condition damages a person's memory and mental processing abilities. In order to do most things in life it is necessary to consult memory.

The memory system is like a giant super-sophisticated filing cabinet with different sections. A person receives and assesses information. If it is important it will be filed away in long-term memory – close relatives' phone numbers, where you went on holiday, the feelings you experienced when your first child was born, what your favourite kind of dinner consists of and what it tastes like, bits of favourite films and countless other things – facts, dislikes, emotional hurts, how to perform particular actions and so on. The amount of available space in the long-term memory appears to be unlimited. People with dementia will tend to remember things from further back in their lives simply because the information was stored when their memory systems were functioning efficiently. Powerful emotional incidents and poems or other things learned by rote seem to last the longest.

There is also a section in the memory for less important things: who you met at the shops yesterday, what you had for dinner last night, a routine visit from a friend or health professional that afternoon. When people are well, it is generally quick and easy for them to retrieve such information; the process is virtually automatic and occurs in split seconds. However, when a person has dementia, this kind of short-term or recent memory is usually the first to be adversely affected as a result of the way dementia impairs a person's ability to store and recall information; it can result in immense frustration.

Even a simple question involves a great deal of mental processing and memory consultation. If a friend texts a straightforward question like 'Fancy going for a drink at the King's Arms after work?' you have to formulate a reply. This involves:

◆ Recognizing the words the other person has used.

◆ Matching them to images stored in your brain of a pub, a glass of wine, the King's Arms, etc.

◆ Assessing how you feel – tired, keen to chat or undecided but persuadable.

◆ Thinking about the logistics of getting to the pub.

◆ Considering if you have enough time.

◆ Wondering what your partner will think, based on how often you have been going out recently.

And much more besides.

Having done all that, you have to make a decision and then respond to the text. This involves consulting your memory, partly consciously and partly automatically. It involves complex mental processing:

- How will I word my reply?
- How do I operate my mobile phone?
- How long should I stay in the pub?
- What will the parking be like?
- What will I do about food?

And so on.

For people who do not have dementia these processes will happen within split seconds, with only a small amount of conscious thought. If any bits of information have been forgotten, strategies will quickly be deployed to find the answer, to sort it out. For a person with dementia, an apparently straightforward series of actions of this sort is a potential minefield. And this is just one simple example.

The whole process is mysterious and unimaginably complex. In the case of a person with dementia some of the links along the way have been damaged. It might be that if they hear 'tomato' they get an image of an apple. Perhaps the correct image appears briefly before vanishing too soon for processing. The negative possibilities are endless and people are affected in many different ways.

Communication between people is like a two-way road but for the person with dementia there are hidden potholes and parts of the road which have completely subsided.

Part of your challenge is to learn where the obstacles are and find ways to help the person get round them.

The above example about going to the pub relates to conversation. However, the problem lies with the memory and with mental processing generally, so that all areas of receptive and expressive communication are affected. A person might recognize a friend of fifty years but be completely incapable of putting a name to the face; they might see their daughter and think it is their late wife. A person might mistake one smell for another or be unable to remember how to carry out a simple task – operating a microwave oven, for instance – which they did with ease in the past.

The difficulties become more severe as the condition progresses. It is sad but inevitable.

In order to help a person achieve the best possible level of communication, a good starting point is to put yourself in their place.

Try to imagine what it would be like gradually to lose the ability to communicate as you have always done in the past – and no doubt taken for granted.

A few years ago I lived in France for a time and I think this experience increased my ability to empathize with what people with dementia go through. I could speak the language reasonably well, but a lot of things that people said still went over my head. Sometimes I would hear a sentence and catch a few key words. Before I could figure it out, the conversation had moved on to something else and then I was faced with the daunting task of trying to interrupt and ask for particular points to be repeated and explained – all in French. Sometimes I ended up missing important bits of information and was left feeling frustrated and powerless.

I did not have dementia, however, and was able to work at improving my French. I also had supportive and understanding friends who did what they could to console and encourage me and help me make progress; any negative feelings I had about my abilities were thus greatly reduced.

A person with dementia needs this kind of help, too.

But the help they need relates to accessing and working with the memory they already have and, in general, not learning new things – whether they be facts and figures or physical activities.

New learning is very hard for a person with dementia; as the condition progresses it becomes to all intents and purposes impossible. In my view, although there may be exceptions in the early stages, any new learning should generally be avoided. It requires a level of mental-processing ability that a person with dementia will not have – and trying to carry out such tasks will almost certainly be stressful.

That said, there are some areas where new learning can occur quite naturally. A person who has carers coming in regularly will soon learn which ones they feel most comfortable with. They might also improve at simple games involving, for instance, throwing balls at targets. But such examples are very different from trying to learn activities which involve the exercise of more complex mental powers, such as the rules of a new card game or following an unusual recipe.

The aim should be to reduce the load placed on a person's mental powers. Why put them under pressure and give them tasks they are no longer equipped to do?

When I worked as a speech and language therapist, I often felt uneasy about the fact that I was expected to carry out assessments of people with dementia. These assessments involved things like showing people pictures of objects and asking them to name them, drawing a clock face to show a particular time, thinking of as many animals as possible in sixty seconds and so on. I clearly remember the look of fear and anxiety on the faces of people as they tried and failed to carry out the exercises. I think assessments of this kind are unavoidable as part of the process of getting a diagnosis or a probable diagnosis, but far harder to justify thereafter.

There is a view that it is good to come up with exercises to stretch a person's brain on the 'use-it-or-lose-it' principle. This might involve simple crosswords or other word games. This can be appropriate but only if the exercises are not too hard – which can be demotivating – and if participating in such activities accords with the person's clearly stated wishes.

In general, I think the aim should be to make life pleasant and stimulating for people whilst at the same time keeping stress and anxiety levels as low as possible.

Although a diagnosis or probable diagnosis can generate positive feelings in a person such as defiance or a determination to find ways to slow down the progress of the condition, I think that many experience very alarming feelings as the condition progresses. There will be few who do not have some of the following emotional responses: anger, apprehension, embarrassment, panic, frustration, denial, loss of confidence, depression, fear of loss of control and of being a burden, as well as a sense of despair and hopelessness.

THE IMPACT AND PROGRESSIVE NATURE OF DEMENTIA

When things happen in the life of a person who does not have dementia, they can make overall sense of them, relate them to past events in their personal history, put them in their place and move on. This is far harder for a person with dementia; perhaps the worst feeling of all is a creeping loss of identity. Auguste Deter, a woman treated by Dr Alois Alzheimer more than a century ago, said she had 'lost herself'. A diagnosis of cancer or motor neurone disease can be hard to come to terms with, but there does appear to be something particularly frightening about a condition that attacks the brain and can appear to result in a loss of self.

Every person has a vast number of memories of varying importance stored in their brains. Once pieces start disappearing or cease to be accessible, it can seem as if the person you know so well is fading away. It is hardly surprising that some people with dementia can become quite rigid about how they want things done or how they behave: they are probably trying to cling on to things that are familiar. These developments can be upsetting. However, even in the much later stages, try to look for and value the memories that do survive – little mannerisms, quirky facial expressions, appreciation of music or pets; all of these are vital parts of the person which will survive for almost the whole of their life.

You should aim to make a person's life as unchallenging yet as agreeable and satisfying as possible. This can be achieved in many ways but the best possible communication with them is a crucial element in trying to help a person retain their identity, their sense of being a valuable and valued person, for the longest time possible.

One important point to bear in mind, however, is this: dementia does not stand still.

It is a progressive condition and a person will gradually deteriorate – even though there might be reasonably long spells when things remain stable. This will happen in different ways for different people with different types of dementia. You should discuss developments regularly with the health professionals involved in the care of the person in order to be as well informed as possible about how things are likely to progress. It is important to be aware of the changes that take place so that you can make adjustments to the way you interact with the person. Things which might have worked well in the early stages might become too difficult, and more importantly, demoralizing, for a person in the more advanced stages.

Bear in mind, too, that apart from the progress of their dementia, the person will also have to contend with the challenges of normal ageing. They might have other specific conditions, Parkinson's disease for example, which can affect muscle movement, which in turn can interfere with the ability to speak clearly.

Some writers have identified as many as ten stages of dementia. I think this is of questionable value: a person does not wake up one day having moved from stage five to stage six overnight. That said, in broad terms I do think it is realistic and useful to be aware that as the condition progresses things do change and you will have to adjust your expectations of what a person will be able to do.

THE THREE MAIN STAGES OF DEMENTIA

Broadly speaking there are three main stages to be aware of – all have a bearing on communication.

Early stages

◆ Some difficulty finding words, particularly those of a more uncommon nature.

◆ Saying the wrong word for something – pineapple instead of banana, for example.

◆ Losing the thread of conversations.

◆ Difficulty following the plot of television dramas.

◆ Being generally forgetful.

◆ Getting up to do something and then forgetting what it was.

◆ Poor short-term memory.

◆ Easily distracted.

◆ Lack of coherence when describing something.

◆ Repeating things said a short time previously.

It can sometimes be hard to differentiate between the effects of dementia and normal ageing in the earliest stages. However, as time goes by, and health professionals become involved and carry out various assessments, the picture becomes clearer and a diagnosis or a probable diagnosis will be given.

As part of the more enlightened approach to dementia nowadays, I think a person has a right to know about their condition and be involved in discussions concerning their diagnosis and treatment. They will almost certainly realize something is wrong and should not be kept in the dark – as might well have happened in the past.

This topic could well be one of your early communicative challenges – helping to explain what the health professionals say and also to ensure that the person's questions and concerns are articulated and answered. Apart from anything else, by being open about things you may well help to reduce a person's understandable anxiety when trying to come to terms with the reality of a life-diminishing condition. Needless to say, any such conversations should be handled with great sensitivity.

That said, there are people who would rather not know, or at least be told as little as possible, and this should of course be respected – everybody is different.

However, there will inevitably be meetings with health professionals from time to time when the subject is likely to be discussed.

This can be an especially difficult and demoralizing time; inevitably a person is likely to have a lot of negative thoughts about the future and your task will be to communicate a positive message whilst at the same time not giving the person unrealistic hope. Whilst I favour openness, I think there can also be arguments in favour of being economical with the truth, particularly when it comes to dealing with questions about what the later stages of dementia can be like. You can justify this to yourself, though – you have no idea how long the person will live. Perhaps they will die of something else before the later stages of dementia are reached.

Any discussion should accentuate the positive:

◆ There is no reason why a person should not lead a fulfilling life for a long time.

◆ The condition is better understood now than in the past.

◆ Many experts are coming up with new ways to make life easier for a person with dementia.

◆ Support, family or otherwise, is available.

◆ Advances have been made in drug treatment.

For as long as possible, people with dementia should be consulted about any adaptations which are being considered for their home – explanatory signs on doors or cupboards, or the creation of memory albums, for instance – all of which are dealt with in detail in later chapters. Even though you might think there is a need for such things, the person might feel that such measures – which they could find embarrassing – are not yet necessary; so far as possible their views should be respected.

It is important to remember that the person with dementia is just that – a person, with rights to express views on matters of relevance to them. That said, as time goes on there is no doubt that you will be required to take unilateral action and make changes in order to keep the person safe and also to make communication of all kinds as straightforward, stimulating and effective as possible. As with most things in life, there is a balance to be struck, which will require careful judgement on your part. It will not always be easy.

In the early stages the person will almost certainly be aware that things are going wrong and might try to disguise the fact. By being open about the condition and helping to make things easier for them you will take pressure off them to pretend that things are all right when they are not.

I remember one woman who told me that when she went to social events she would make a point of never talking to anyone for more than a minute or two before moving on. In this way she was able to stick to social pleasantries – 'Nice to see you', 'How's the family?', 'Terrible weather recently', and so on.

She knew that if she became more engaged with a fellow guest her difficulties were likely to be exposed.

Middle stages

◆ Finding it harder to understand things that are said to them unless they are straightforward and familiar.

◆ Increasing use of 'empty' words and phrases, for example 'thingummy', 'one of them things', 'over there'. This will usually happen because the person's word-finding difficulties have become more acute.

◆ Increasing difficulties with reading.

◆ Difficulty carrying out everyday tasks – making a cup of tea, operating the remote control – which would have been easy before.

◆ Less comfortable meeting new people and dealing with unfamiliar situations.

◆ Innocently relating events which are partially or totally untrue as if they are fact.

◆ In conversation, sometimes forgetting the right word and using another random word to fill the gap.

◆ Coming out with 'words' that are not in fact words at all.

◆ Difficulty with reasoning.

◆ Facial expressiveness begins to decline; fewer and less rich facial reactions.

◆ Difficulty at times understanding what a person says. Those who are with the person learn how to make sense of what they say and might need to 'interpret' for others.

◆ Apart from impaired use of language, the person might also speak quietly or indistinctly and be less and less able to observe the norms of everyday conversation.

Later stages

◆ Might make little sense when speaking.

◆ Difficulty understanding what is said, even if it is very straightforward.

◆ Using bad language or being rude or aggressive – even someone who has rarely behaved like this in the past.

◆ Difficulty in carrying out the simplest tasks.

◆ Repeating what others say back to them without really understanding the words.

◆ Communicating non-verbally to a greater degree.

◆ Talking about the past as if it is the present – and perhaps mistaking you for another close relative or not recognizing you at all.

Eventually the condition will adversely affect every aspect of life.

Don't forget that a person in the early stages often retains a considerable level of mental ability, and to treat them as if they were in the middle stages might well make them feel patronized or worse. It might simply be a case of discreetly monitoring the person and intervening only if there is a specific need.

Similarly, a person in the middle stages or beyond cannot be expected to attempt ways of communicating that are now beyond them. This will simply set them up to fail and this in turn will almost certainly contribute to negative feelings or even depression.

As the journey progresses, the person will gradually have less and less insight into their condition and greatly reduced awareness of events in the world around them. However, even in the much later stages there will be a smile, a look, a gesture in response to something you say or something the person sees or hears that will make you realize that they are still there. The better you are able to communicate with them in whatever ways work, the more often you will be able to enjoy these glimpses.

3

Creating the Best Environment for Good Communication

Dementia diminishes a person's ability to communicate as a result of its impact on many aspects of brain function. It follows, therefore, that every single thing that is associated with the communicative process should be made as easy and smooth as possible. This will give the person the best possible opportunity to use to the full the capacity they retain.

Of course not all of the following points will apply to everybody, and in the early to middle stages the person might well continue to attend to many of them with little or no help from you.

HEARING
As part of the normal ageing process everybody's hearing becomes less sharp. Hearing deficits beyond normal ageing will have an increasingly negative impact on a person's ability to communicate because – at the risk of stating the obvious – they will not always make out everything that is said. They will also be more likely to mishear words, 'red' instead of 'fed', for instance. They might ask for things to be repeated constantly. At times they might just stop trying to keep up and end up feeling excluded.

There are a number of questions you should ask if you suspect that a person is experiencing hearing difficulties.

1. Has there been a recent assessment by an audiologist?

2. Have the person's ears been checked for a build-up of wax recently?

3. If a person has hearing aids, do they work properly; do they need new batteries?

4. Can the person actually operate the hearing aids reliably? Even for people who do not have dementia, hearing aids are notoriously finicky.

In addition, it is important to do what you can to ensure the aids do not go missing – a common problem. Here are some points to bear in mind on this subject:

◈ The best way to make sure aids do not fall out is to ensure that they are correctly fitted in the first place. People with dementia might not be able to do this reliably and so might need discreet assistance and monitoring.

◈ Be aware of any activities, for example going up and down stairs, eating, etc., that seem to be associated with the aids coming out.

◈ If possible, have a spare set of hearing aids.

◈ As well as reducing a person's ability to hear, a build-up of ear wax can make it more difficult to fit hearing aids snugly.

◈ It is possible to obtain sticky pads and other accessories such as retainers, which can help to ensure that the hearing aids stay in place.

You should consult an appropriate adviser if you come across problems you can't deal with yourself. In addition, the website for Action on Hearing Loss (formerly the Royal National Institute for Deaf People) contains a great deal of useful information.

VISION

Vision is a particularly important communication channel. Apart from the ability to see things, eyesight helps a person to 'hear' better by reading non-verbal communication such as facial expressions and body language. Everybody's eyesight deteriorates as the years roll by. This is true for people with dementia, too – but they might not think to tell you that it is happening. Accordingly it is necessary to be proactive:

◆ Carry out discreet informal assessments now and then by asking the person to read a small headline in their newspaper or pass you a small object.

◆ Give gentle prompts to put glasses on at appropriate times if the person does not do it.

◆ Ensure glasses are cleaned regularly, preferably daily, to remove any dirt that might reduce clarity.

◆ Consider getting a cord for the glasses so that they are less likely to be lost. Ensure there is a spare pair of glasses available.

◆ Consider getting a pair of glasses with tinted glass to avoid glare during sunny spells.

◆ Ensure a person's glasses have the right prescription by arranging eye tests with an optician from time to time.

◆ An optician can also assess and advise on other matters which might have a bearing on eyesight, such as irritable eye conditions, as well as more serious diseases such as glaucoma.

◆ As a general rule a person whose vision has deteriorated will find it easier to see things where there are marked colour contrasts.

And don't forget – communication is a two-way process – make sure that you attend to your own hearing and sight.

PHYSICAL ISSUES

Posture

Good posture helps to ensure good voice production. Vocal sounds are produced with air that comes up from the lungs, past the larynx and out through the mouth. If a person is slouching or has a drooping head then the power of their air supply will be reduced and their voice can become weak and quiet. A person might be barely audible and this will make any kind of conversational exchange difficult – particularly with a visitor who does not know the person well.

In addition, in more extreme cases, the person's ability to see what is going on in a room could be restricted. They might only be able to see another person's lower half. The effort of trying to see more might cause muscle or eye strain.

If the person's physical condition makes it difficult to achieve a reasonably good posture, adaptations should be made:

◆ Kneel on the floor when talking to the person.

◆ Don't approach them from the side or behind.

◆ Place newspapers or photographs at a low level – to reduce the effort the person has to make to see all of them.

Aim to achieve the best, most upright, posture that is reasonably and comfortably possible for a person. To an extent this is common sense, but a physiotherapist will be able to provide specific advice where necessary.

Pain

Sometimes a person with dementia experiences pain but, particularly in the later stages, cannot find the necessary words to explain what is wrong. You will have to develop good observational skills and a knack for finding ways to encourage them to express what is going on, and then take appropriate action by giving medication or calling the doctor. Clearly, if a person is in any kind of pain or discomfort this will be a distraction that will make any kind of communicative activity less likely to be successful. Similarly, a person should ideally have had sufficient sleep and not be hungry or thirsty.

Lack of energy

Lack of energy is not uncommon among older people generally; this makes any kind of activity effortful. Being indoors in a warm stuffy environment tends to make this worse – although the person should not feel cold. Accordingly, try to ensure that the person gets some fresh air on a regular basis. Apart from the obvious health benefits, a change of scene can be stimulating and provide opportunities to see things that can spark conversation.

Oral hygiene

Oral hygiene is very important. With the best will in the world, any form of communicative activity will be made less appealing if a person has bad breath. This is true of grooming generally. If a person emits unpleasant smells from their mouth, has unkempt hair and wears stained clothes, visitors will be discouraged from coming back – and the person with dementia will be the loser.

In addition, with poor oral hygiene a person might develop ulcers or other sores which could make the act of speaking painful or uncomfortable. The danger is that rather than attempt to say anything the person just clams up. Even if they do not, the quality of their language production might be adversely affected so that what they do say is less distinct.

Take medical or dental advice sooner rather than later.

You should ensure that if a person has dentures, they are kept clean and fit well. Poorly fitting dentures which move around in the mouth make it harder for the person to speak and harder for people to hear clearly what they are saying. As a person ages there can be small changes in the physical structure of the mouth which result in dentures not fitting as well as they did in the past and new ones might be required.

A person with dementia might forget to go to the toilet or simply not read the signs soon enough. Physical discomfort will hamper the chances of good communication and so – if this is an issue – you should try to be aware of when the person last went to the toilet and give gentle reminders from time to time.

ALCOHOL

If a person has been in the habit of enjoying a glass of wine or beer then there is no reason why this should not continue – unless it creates specific problems such as interference with sleep patterns. If you are in any doubt check with the person's doctor. Alcohol has been associated with conviviality and conversation since time immemorial and this is not something that should be stopped just because a person has dementia. A moderate amount can enhance communication; as the condition advances, supervision will be required.

ROOMS AND PHYSICAL SPACE

A person with dementia, particularly later on, will probably spend a lot of time in a small amount of space, most likely a living room and a bedroom. These areas should be as well suited as possible to facilitating communication.

Avoid unnecessary clutter. It is a good idea to have some familiar pictures on the walls and some souvenirs on the mantelpiece in order to personalize rooms, especially the bedroom, but don't overdo it. If the room is crowded with things this can be over-stimulating and distracting; try to strike a reasonable balance and choose things that reflect the person's tastes.

Another point is that the person might have reduced mobility and will therefore appreciate a room that is easy to navigate, with few obstructions – and of course this will make the room safer.

The last thing you want is a person looking out from their chair thinking, 'How do I get out of here?'

A few well-placed solid and secure pieces of furniture to lean against can also be helpful for coming and going.

While a person with dementia is sitting in their chair, it will be reassuring for them to see the same bits of furniture in the same places with the same pictures on the wall; the message transmitted is one of continuity. Avoid constant change, which will result in a person having to learn to adjust to new layouts. This is not to say that there can be no change but that it should generally be in minor details, say a postcard or a bunch of flowers; and any such changes should be drawn to the person's attention.

Keep the room well lit during the day when a person might be looking at pictures or a newspaper. Windows should be kept clean to allow the maximum amount of light in. If the lighting is dingy it makes it harder to see things, not least the subtleties of facial expressions. At night, avoid having too many shadows in the room. In the later stages in particular, a person with dementia can mistake shadows for mysterious and alarming shapes, which they might see as unknown or threatening people.

There is some anecdotal evidence that simple pastel colours are the most peaceful and relaxing, although whatever the colours, the environment should include contrasts. As with much else it will depend on the preferences of the particular person. If possible, carpets and floor coverings should be plain. It is possible for people in the later stages of dementia to be confused by complex patterns and they might see a floor covering with black shapes as a series of holes in the ground. There has even been a reported instance of a man with dementia viewing some large white shapes in a carpet as urinals, with unfortunate consequences.

Keep rooms clean and tidy as you would for yourself. If you think it is not so important because the person will not notice, you will be giving out the message that they deserve less consideration.

When setting the table for meals, invest some time and effort in making it look interesting and colourful. In this way you will be indicating that the person is valued and deserves thoughtful treatment. You might not get any thanks from the person you are looking after – it often goes with the condition – but it is always better to be sending out positive signals.

Some more points to bear in mind about mealtimes:

Provide a varied range of food. This should consist of dishes the person has long been familiar with – this sends a message of continuity. It is probably not a good idea to introduce the exotic new recipes you saw on the television.

Ensure that the tablecloth, plates, mats, cutlery and food feature strongly contrasting colours. This has been found helpful, as not eating enough can be an issue for people with dementia. Fish in white sauce on a pale plate will be difficult to see. Everything should be done to make mealtimes as straightforward as possible.

Consider the seating arrangement. A person who has started to experience difficulty using cutlery might benefit from being placed opposite – and thus able to observe – a person who has no such difficulty.

Help the person in making a choice. If a person spends a lot of time in bed and regularly has breakfast in bed, it can be cumbersome to offer a reasonable degree of choice other than by explaining what is on offer verbally – which might be confusing. To help with this, you could try cutting out the fronts of some cereal or biscuit packets or yoghurt cartons and take them through to them.

Try to make sure the person understands what is for lunch or dinner. Do this just before or as it is being served, rather than simply putting a plate of food down in front of them.

Provide a range of healthy finger foods. In the later stages, a person might find it increasingly difficult to use cutlery – so you might want to consider finger food, which could help to preserve independence. On a subliminal level, finger food communicates the message that eating can continue to be enjoyable and need not involve much thought or planning.

Think about the positioning of the chair the person usually sits in. This can be important. You could have the person facing a wall or you could make things much more interesting by having them face a window with some kind of a view, perhaps a street scene with some human activity. Particularly in the later stages, this could be a way of providing stimulation and interest at a time when a person might be less mobile.

Create a pleasant and welcoming environment. As part of this overall aim, consider having some agreeable aromas where the person regularly sits: scented candles, fresh coffee, or perhaps fresh cut flowers – whatever you think they would appreciate most, based on your knowledge of them. Such aromas or scents might spark off agreeable memories or feelings. Bear in mind, however, that a person's tastes can change and the fact that someone liked something years before is not a guarantee that they still do. Part of the skill you develop should be to routinely monitor such things.

Consider having things that are pleasant to handle near the person – a bowl containing pieces of silk, those little meditation balls you roll around in your hand which make pleasant sounds, bean bags or smooth wooden ornaments.

Watch out for mirrors. They can be useful and add depth to a room. However, you have to think about whether a person with dementia wants constant reminders of their declining appearance. Also, in the later stages, the person might have difficulty understanding that it is their own reflection they see and might be confused or even alarmed by what they perceive to be a stranger in the room.

Try to keep extraneous noise to a minimum. If possible, do washing or vacuuming when a person is least likely to be disturbed by it. In particular, try to avoid such distractions when any specific activities are going to take place. People with dementia can be particularly sensitive to a whole range of sounds that other people would not find especially distracting. Clearly you have no control over police sirens or aircraft, but there are many ways to rejig the life of the house to create quieter spells.

Do your best to arrange the room with the person in mind.

Why not sit in the person's chair for a few minutes when they are out of the room. Just think about everything from their perspective and see if there are any beneficial changes that could be made.

If the weather is favourable, set something up outside – if there is access to a garden (or other outdoor space such as a balcony or a roof terrace). A garden provides a whole range of opportunities for pleasing communion with the outside world, from watching birds (make sure there are some well-filled feeders around the garden), trees and clouds to observing the general bustle of life in the street. Draw the person's attention to things of interest that might stimulate conversation.

Remember that a person with dementia will always prefer an environment that is calm and where things happen quietly and at a moderate pace. This allows them to adjust and reduces the risk that they will be alarmed or taken by surprise by unexpected sounds.

Finally, although you know that in reality a great deal has changed in your relationship with the person, try as far as possible to keep things as they were in the past. You are now helping to care for the person, but try also to continue being the close relative or friend you have always been.

ROUTINES

You should aim to have the same things – meals, taking a bath, going to the shops, watching television programmes, whatever

– at similar times and in similar ways each day. When memory is no longer working efficiently, it is reassuring for a person to have daily patterns which don't change much; they will appreciate solid foundations.

EQUIPMENT AND TECHNOLOGY

Try to ensure that any pieces of equipment a person continues to use are as straightforward as possible. Obvious examples are telephones, mobile or fixed, and television controls. You should have newer models that have large buttons and minimal controls. There are many such phones on the market. Any old ones should be disposed of or put out of sight in a drawer. Having several lying around the place and expecting the person to be able to remember, or work out, which is the right one is likely to cause confusion and frustration. There are new laptops and tablets coming on to the market (one example is Samsung's *Breezie*) that feature very straightforward on-screen commands – for making video calls, for instance.

There is no reason why a person with dementia should not be able to telephone and receive calls from relatives and friends for a considerable length of time. For people who live alone, in particular, a telephone can be a vital line of communication.

And it is a good idea to phone the person yourself from time to time – partly to stay in touch or give reminders about, for example, taking pills, and partly to assess their current level of ability to use the phone.

Make sure that the numbers used most often are stored as speed dials; it is possible also to include photographs of people to be called. Details of the relevant numbers and the people they relate to, along with clear and simple instructions, should be printed in large-size font on an A4 sheet of paper, laminated (preferably) and put up on the wall close to the landline. Don't put it in a drawer or leave it loose on top of a table where it might get lost or hidden.

There will eventually come a time when using any equipment will become too difficult for a person with more advanced dementia; you have to be realistic about this. You should probably remove items like mobile phones from view.

Advances in technology are resulting in many more products coming onto the market which, although not specifically aimed at people with dementia, have great potential to make aspects of their lives easier and safer – especially those who live on their own. For instance there are monitoring systems that involve placing sensors around the house which are linked to external devices such as mobile phones or tablets. The 'remote carer' – i.e. you – can thus tell, for instance, if a person has got up in the morning, cooked a meal, forgotten to switch off a tap or left the back door open. If the person goes out, the system allows you to know when and at what time they return. It might all be a bit like Big Brother, but devices of this sort have the potential to enable a person to stay at home safely for longer.

There are even small robots (sometimes referred to as home care robots), which can carry out some of the functions of carers, such as reminding them to have a meal. Such devices are still very uncommon (and expensive) but might become more popular as governments struggle to cope with the costs of providing care for people with dementia and seek to enable people to remain in their own homes. That said, small robots moving around the house could be confusing and alarming for some.

MAIL

The arrival of a letter explaining new gas charges or setting out the following year's council tax can be hard for anybody to follow – but much harder for a person with dementia. Also they might put bills away somewhere and then forget where.

It is a tricky subject. You could get all mail redirected to you or someone else – but the person might feel that they are being treated like a child by having this part of their life suddenly taken away from them. As an alternative you could consider the following:

1. Make sure as many payments as possible are made by direct debit and have bank statements sent to you. (This might involve you becoming an attorney for the person; this topic is dealt with in Chapter 11.)

2. Make arrangements with legal or tax advisers that you are copied into any correspondence, so that you are prepared for a phone call from the person about a letter.

3. Encourage the person to put all mail received – unopened – into one obvious place, perhaps a drawer near the letter box – and then go through it all with them when you visit. Alternatively, you could go over the mail by phone – but this will be more difficult.

UNSOLICITED PHONE CALLS AND VISITS TO THE HOUSE

The danger here is that the person with dementia gets entangled with somebody trying to sell something.

So far as unsolicited phone calls are concerned there are online services which enable you to register the person's number as belonging to someone who does not wish to receive unsolicited phone calls. This will not stop all calls but it should cut them down substantially.

Encourage the person to use a stock phrase for any calls that do get through, for example: 'My husband/son/daughter/social worker handles these things on my behalf. Send a letter if you wish.' This should be printed out and placed near the phone and/or front door.

Problems can also arise with people visiting the house trying to sell things or getting a person to sign direct debit forms, in favour of a particular charity for instance. It is not hard to imagine how difficult situations like this are for many people with dementia. The consequences can be serious if they do agree to take on financial obligations. If the person lives alone then the best course is probably to put a sign on the door saying that unsolicited visitors are prohibited. You could perhaps also include your own mobile number for anyone who wishes to discuss the matter. They almost certainly won't.

CHOOSING THE RIGHT MOMENT FOR COMMUNICATIVE ACTIVITIES

Whenever you are going to engage in any kind of communicative activity, other than routine everyday stuff, you want to make sure that the conditions are as favourable as possible. Remember that one of the skills you need to develop is thinking ahead, a bit like a chauffeur who wants to make a journey as smooth as possible, without sudden braking or unexpected U-turns. After a while this will become automatic.

Be aware of a person's drug regime. There might be times when they will be drowsy. The doctor should advise you on such side effects. Time of day can be important. After lunch a person might not be at their most alert. Similarly, a person might be quite slow to get going in the morning. You want them to be as receptive as possible.

PREPARING FOR OUTINGS AND APPOINTMENTS

From time to time a person will have appointments with the doctor, dentist, optician, etc. In addition there will be times when you go out on visits to friends or interesting places. The appointments are necessary and the outings can provide an agreeable experience. However, such events, which disrupt the everyday rhythms and patterns of life, can be unsettling for a person with dementia, particularly in the later stages. Accordingly, you need to use good communication techniques to prepare the ground.

One key question is when do you tell the person? A week in advance? No good. Far too long. Chances are they will have forgotten about it not long after you told them. A few minutes beforehand? Is that really giving them enough time to absorb the fact? There is no correct answer here.

If the event is going to happen in the afternoon it will probably be best to mention it firstly in the morning, as part of laying the ground. You could then mention it again after lunch. A short time before you will be departing, say half an hour, you should appear holding the person's coat or bag or gloves and say that you will be leaving soon for the appointment/outing you talked about earlier. By holding an outdoor item in this way, you will be providing a visual cue that backs up what you are saying.

Be aware of the person's response. If they become agitated and it is clear – once they have understood the nature of the outing – that they do not want to participate, then you have to decide how important the event in question is. If it is a walk in the park, it is almost certainly best to accept the message they are sending and forget the outing. If, however, it is a doctor's appointment, you will have to decide whether it can be postponed or not.

All such matters will depend to a large extent on how far advanced the condition is.

FORMING AN INFORMAL SUPPORT NETWORK

You should put together an informal team of people made up of those who will most regularly be in contact with the person, and a few others who can help from time to time. I am using the word 'team' in a very loose sense. It is really about you having a clear idea of who you might be able to call on in particular situations. The people themselves might well be unaware that you think of them in this way. It is hard to be specific because every family situation will be different. Some people find that they have a lot of people living nearby who are willing to get involved, others don't. You really just have to play the hand you are dealt.

You will usually be the main contact. It will be for you or someone on your behalf to communicate with people in the team, to explain difficulties or to request help. It is a vital advocacy role. The person with dementia will probably struggle to initiate such communication.

It follows that in approaching the care of a person with dementia you will need, or need to develop, good communication skills for dealing with a variety of people and not just the person with dementia.

Such skills will involve understanding as well as possible what problems a person is experiencing and making sure that a health professional, or whoever, clearly understands them too. This role will be particularly important when it comes to trying to explain physical symptoms a person is experiencing.

Let's say you are the son of a widow who has dementia, you live a few doors away from her and see her most days. You have a brother who lives a three-hour drive away and a sister who lives abroad. You hope that your brother will visit fairly regularly and that your sister will stay in touch via Skype and visit when she can. All three of you will have discussions when any important decisions have to be made.

One point to stress here is that while it is essential to make relatives and friends aware of matters of importance concerning the person with dementia, this should never happen in the presence of the person.

I am horrified when I see interviews with carers taking place on television while their father or mother or husband or wife (with dementia) sits next to them, silent and expressionless. The carer answers all sorts of highly personal questions about the impact of the condition on their lives and sometimes become tearful. Who knows what the person with dementia sitting there makes of it all? Perhaps they are not upset, but what if they are and are unable to express this? No, any information that you want to give to other people should – so far as practically possible – be imparted when you are not in the presence or hearing of the person with dementia.

Here are some examples of additional people you could include in the team:

Other close relatives who live within easy reach. You should be prepared to call on them to help with particular tasks or to cover for you when you are unavailable. You should make them aware of the situation as it develops and brief them about some basic communication guidelines.

Old friends who are happy to be involved. Those who do make themselves available can provide invaluable companionship and opportunities for conversation and reminiscence. Try to set up reasonably regular visits.

Healthcare professionals. These can include, for instance, GP, district nurse, social worker, occupational therapist, speech and language therapist, physiotherapist and, in the UK, an Admiral Nurse. Admiral Nurses specialize in the care and support of people with dementia and their families. You should have all contact details near at hand. You should be aware of what each of these professionals can do to help and not hesitate to contact them should the need arise.

Religious organizations. If a person has been in the habit of attending church or other religious establishments, this will have provided them with an important form of communication both in terms of worship and also meeting like-minded people. Similarly, the person might have been a member of a club which involved regular meetings or group activities.

Talk to the minister or organizer. The hope is that the person in charge – once the situation is explained to them – will be sympathetic and prepared to make changes or allowances which will permit the person to be involved for as long as possible.

Neighbours. They might or might not be part of the team, but either way you should consider having a discreet word to make them aware of the situation. They may well have worked it out already. Some might be only too pleased to offer to help in various ways. Others will look the other way.

Depending on your personality, you might find that initiating all of this, and having to be quite assertive at times, will take you out of your comfort zone. Always try to remember that what you are doing could help the person with dementia. Bear in mind, too, that people are often happy to help – but they do need to be asked.

4

Talking and Conversation

Although communication in the broadest sense goes far beyond spoken words and conversation, they do nonetheless constitute a very important element of communicating with a person with dementia. As time goes by, though, conversation will become less rich. There will be less vocabulary, less skilful development of arguments, more chopping and changing of topics.

You will of course recognize what has been lost but that is now in the past and you have to let it go – and not continue to try to get the person to recapture the old ways of conversing. This will only lead to stress and frustration. This is all part of recasting your approach to communication.

TALKING TO SOMEONE WITH DEMENTIA

If you meet up with a friend you might have an idea of a few things you want to discuss or you might just start things off by saying, 'So what's been happening?' Either way, you will soon be chatting away nineteen to the dozen. When you talk to a person with dementia things are different; it is a good idea to have some kind of conversational plan – an idea of topics that are likely to work best. There is more information on this particular aspect of communication in Chapter 5.

In order to facilitate verbal communication of every kind there are a number of guidelines to bear in mind. Their relevance will vary according to the person as well as their stage in the dementia journey. You should ensure that what you expect of a person is within their current capability. While of course you respect the person and treat them as an equal, the truth is that you will sometimes have to engage in a little subterfuge and manipulation. You will deploy strategies and tactics in order to make things happen in the most suitable way.

You should not worry about this, as long as whatever you do, you do with respect and consideration, in the best interests of the person.

Bear in mind, too, that conversation with a person with dementia will almost invariably require more effort and energy than would be the case if you were having a relaxing chat with a friend over a glass of wine. Don't be surprised or resentful about this.

Whatever you do, keep the amount of mental processing required of the person – consulting memory, reasoning, explaining and understanding – to a minimum.

Before saying anything, make sure you have the person's attention. You can do this by:

◆ Saying their name.
◆ Being at the same level as them.
◆ Gently touching their arm.
◆ Making good eye contact.
◆ Allowing them time to tune in.

The whole process might only take a few seconds but it will prepare the ground.

Here is an example of how you might propose an outing to a person who is around the middle stages of dementia.

> YOU: 'Mum . . .'
>
> PAUSE. As you make eye contact, smile, touch her arm, tilt head slightly to one side, and ensure you have her attention before proceeding further.
>
> YOU: 'I thought it would be nice to do something together.'
>
> PAUSE. Ensure this idea has registered (Mum might say, 'Oh yes') then move on.
>
> YOU: 'Go and see a film.'
>
> PAUSE. Check this has registered (Mum might say 'That's nice').
>
> YOU: 'I see *Titanic* is on, the big ship that hit the iceberg – you liked that film.'
>
> PAUSE. Look for facial or other reactions that indicate understanding.
>
> YOU: 'Would you like to go and see *Titanic*?'

Note that it is a good idea to move from the more general to the more specific.

This sort of technique is particularly important when you have to carry out any physical manoeuvres in the case of people with physical disabilities or mobility problems. It can also be very helpful for simple daily tasks such as helping the person to get into a bath.

Let's say a person finds it a real effort to get out of a chair but can manage with assistance. Use the above techniques to get the person tuned in and prepared.

> YOU: 'Dad, I'm going to help you up now.'
>
> PAUSE. Ensure this is understood as you slip your arm round him.
>
> YOU: 'Now, I'm going to put my hand under your elbow. All right?'
>
> PAUSE. Look for evidence, a nod, a confirmatory look, then proceed.

In time, this approach will become more natural and semi-automatic. It is, however, important always to remember that anything that requires mental processing takes longer, and increasingly so, for a person with dementia. If you give them that bit of extra time you will make life easier for them and for you.

The important thing from your point of view is to be patient. This might be difficult if you are used to doing things quickly without much active thought – but it will benefit the person.

PREPARING FOR CONVERSATION

Here are some important general points:

◆ Make sure your face is roughly at the same level as the person you are talking to, whether they be standing or sitting. If sitting, lean slightly towards the person to indicate that you are paying attention.

◆ A person with dementia might well be experiencing a degree of agitation and distraction in their lives already – don't add to it by being restless or constantly looking around as you talk.

◆ Put your mobile on silent or switch it off. The sudden sound of the ring tone or a text coming in will be an unwelcome, possibly alarming, distraction for the person.

◆ When you encounter a person after a lapse of time – in the morning, or when you pay a visit – try to assess their general mood and demeanour. If it is clear that they are experiencing a low mood, or tired, do not try to be overly jolly in order to cheer them up. Go in at their level initially, engage, and then see if you can find conversation or activities that might help to lighten the mood.

IMPORTANT POINTS TO OBSERVE DURING CONVERSATION

Avoid the use of unnecessary words
You could say:

'Mum, do you fancy a piece of that apple pie Jane made yesterday – you said you liked it even though it was a bit sweet – I could heat it up and maybe have it with some cream, or I could make some custard. What do you reckon?'

Most people with dementia, certainly those in the middle stages and beyond, would find this hard to follow. They would understand that they are being asked a question, something to do with food, and that they need to make a decision, but mostly they would just be reminded of their failing mental powers. You could make it much easier:

Having made sure you have her attention say:

'Mum . . . apple pie?' Once you have an answer to that say, 'Hot or cold?' and then 'Cream or custard?'

Always think a bit ahead and ask yourself if you can say what you want to say in fewer words. You usually can.

If the phone or doorbell rings, a person with dementia might be alarmed. This unexpected intrusion might generate a range of questions in their minds. Don't say, 'Oh don't worry, it's just the phone.' It is far better to provide a full and logical explanation – if possible. This gives reassurance and an explanation at the moment the issue arises. 'I think that will be Mr Smith the window cleaner, he said he might phone this afternoon.' Confirm the position once you have taken the call.

Similarly, if a person is frustrated by their inability to, say, recall the name of a family pet from the past, you could just dismiss the question: 'It doesn't matter, it's not important.' Far better would be to say, 'He was called Buster. I'll write it down and see if I can find some old photos.'

If you talk at a rate faster than they can process, this will make it difficult for a person with dementia to keep up. Always try to go at their pace or a little slower. This can be hard. The way you are used to conversing, as compared with talking to a person with dementia, is a bit like the difference between driving fast on a motorway versus dawdling along a country road.

The person can't change, so you have to. Pull off the motorway and get behind their car.

Avoid giving orders in a brusque manner

It can be hard to avoid this at times, especially if you are feeling frustrated and close to the end of your tether. However, nobody likes being talked to like that and it will make it harder for the person to gather their thoughts and comply with whatever it is you want them to do. It's the same with criticism – a person with dementia can surely be spared the hurt this can cause.

Try not to override a person's express wishes unless it is unavoidable

If they want to do something and the only reason you have against it is that it will cause you a degree of inconvenience, see if you can find a compromise that allows the person to do what they want whilst at the same time causing least inconvenience to you. Otherwise the message communicated to the person will be that they no longer have the ability to exercise choice. They might well feel as if they are being treated like a child.

For instance, you might have decided to look at old photographs one afternoon, and have gone to some trouble to set everything up in the living room. The person makes it clear that they don't want to do this but would rather go out in the car to the shops, something you were planning to do the following day. If you insist on looking at the photographs, there is a good chance the person will not engage and you will end up having to give up after a while. Far better to change your plans, go to the shops and hope that looking at photographs will be successful on another occasion.

Don't finish a person's sentences for them

Despite the temptation, it is a bad and patronizing communication technique at the best of times; and don't forget that a person with dementia will need extra time to gather their thoughts. Giving gentle cues if the person seems to be losing their thread is, however, fine.

Allow silences; this is very important

It is almost certainly the case that you will be the only one who will feel uncomfortable – as you would if a chatty friend suddenly went quiet for no apparent reason. A person with dementia needs time to formulate what they want to say; and they will become less and less bothered by the demands of social graces, for example the idea that you should always try to keep a conversation going. If there are silences, you should continue to pay attention with eye contact and perhaps slightly raised eyebrows to show that you are available.

This can be quite hard – you probably have a good idea of what the person is wanting to say, might well have heard it many times before and your attention might wander.

You might spend much of your time in a fast-moving world of offices, task-oriented work, emails, texts, and the internet, where communication occurs in split seconds. But you should try to step out of that world and into theirs and let them say things in their own way and in their own time. It is different from how you are used to carrying on a conversation – once more it's a case of all change.

Perhaps, before spending time with a person, you should find a quiet space, breathe deeply and take a few moments to get yourself into the right frame of mind.

Deliver one point at a time

When it is you who is speaking, deliver one point at a time and try to ensure that it has been understood before moving on to the next one. Keep your sentences reasonably short and do not digress. Consider repeating some of the main points by saying them in different ways. The need to do this will increase with the passage of time.

Always remember that the person will probably struggle to retain details of long stories, so avoid these – keep them short and to the point.

The subject of social occasions is touched on elsewhere in the book. They can be very pleasant for a person with dementia, but if there are a few people talking they might well find the conversation hard to follow. You can help in these situations by contributing some brief summaries – spoken directly to the person – to try and keep them connected to what is being discussed: 'John was just telling us about his holiday in Spain.' In addition, discreetly alert the person to changes in topic as they arise.

Visitors with no experience of dementia might, perfectly understandably, direct their conversation to people in the group who do not have dementia – with whom they can have the kind of easy conversation they are used to. Encourage visitors to include the person with dementia – even if this only involves making eye contact from time to time when they are speaking.

If the person is involved in a conversation with two other people try to make sure that they can see the faces of both people as they are talking. Facial expressions give a great many cues, which help to throw light on the words that are being spoken.

When you are conversing with the person, stay close to them; try not to look out of the window, or at your watch, or at some object in the room. In addition, don't move around while you are talking, make sudden movements or hand gestures or, worse still, expect the person to pick up on things you say as you are coming into or going out of a room. Furthermore, don't change the topic of conversation by going off at a tangent about something that suddenly comes into your mind.

All such things will distract or confuse the person and could well mean that what you are saying is far less likely to be understood.

Don't cover your mouth when you are talking. People are used to watching the movement of lips when engaged in conversation.

Use the name of the person you are talking to quite a lot. This will help them to stay engaged in the conversation. Everybody's attention is grabbed by the mention of their own name.

Try to avoid, 'he', 'she', 'it' and 'they' . . . or at least greatly reduce the use of them. You might know instantly who or what is being referred to but a person with dementia might not. 'David went there', not 'He went there' – even if you mentioned David's name a short time before and it seems totally obvious to whom 'he' refers.

Avoid the meaning of times on a clock and make use of events. Do this if it becomes clear that a person no longer understands. For instance, instead of saying 'He's coming at two o' clock', say 'He's coming after lunch.'

Have a few stock phrases for particular situations that happen every day. There are a lot of different ways to tell a person that their midday meal is ready. However, if you use them all randomly then the person will have to tune in each time. 'Time for lunch' accompanied by pointing towards the kitchen might work for you. If it does, stick to it – and the same for going to the shops or getting ready for bed. A few familiar phrases will help to make the transitions easier.

The way you use your voice is important. You should aim to make the way you speak as easy to follow as possible. The following are examples of ways that can help:

◆ Speak clearly.

◆ Speak a little bit more slowly than you would normally.

◆ Speak a little bit louder than you usually do – though this can be stressful for people who have a naturally quiet voice.

◆ Emphasize the key words in what you are saying, but don't overdo it.

None of this is entirely natural and it can result in a slightly stilted way of talking – but it will help to make communication with a person with dementia easier and will come more naturally with practice.

Never apply pressure to a person to give an answer or explain more about what they are saying. This will only result in raised anxiety levels.

In the later stages in particular, you might well be shocked at some of the fundamental things a person forgets – your name, a much-loved pet whose death caused great sorrow at the time. It can be upsetting and very hard to come to terms with this, but it is a direct result of the person's condition.

Don't express surprise or react emotionally in front of the person – 'But of course you know who I am, I'm Laura, your niece.' This will not achieve anything positive. Just remind the person gently and give them time for this to register.

On a different occasion, with different cues, the person might say your name without difficulty – be happy when it happens. You can't change the situation, so you have to accept it without making the person feel inadequate – and move on.

Don't be patronizing. You will be if you say something like, 'There's a good girl, time to go for our bath now.' This is not only patronizing it is also untrue since presumably it is only the person with dementia who is going for a bath. On the other hand, 'We are going to the shops after breakfast' is fine – neither patronizing nor untrue.

Pay good attention when a person is talking. This helps to keep the person on track. You can do this through good eye contact, nods, moderate use of 'uh huh', 'mmmm' and so on, whatever feels right and gives the message that you are still engaged with what the person is saying. Don't overdo it though – if you do, this can result in the person feeling rushed.

Although in principle good eye contact is desirable, there are limits. If you make a laser-like connection without a break, this could feel unsettling or even threatening. It might also be that a woman could find excessive amounts of eye contact from a man intrusive. It is a question of judgement and sensitivity.

In general, humour is a good thing. There is plenty that is very far from amusing about the challenges of caring for a person with dementia, and any opportunities for light relief should be seized with both hands. If something seems funny, respond to it spontaneously and encourage the person to do the same. Don't overdo it, though, otherwise your laughter might come over as insincere.

Note, too, that you should always take great care to avoid any possibility that the person is made to feel that they are being made fun of in any way – that they are the butt of the joke.

The person will probably feel very good about saying something that makes other people laugh and so if they do make an effort to crack a joke, even if it is not that great, do respond as they would like you to – with clear signs of amusement. Simple jokes from childhood might go down well as time goes by.

A little self-deprecating and empathic humour on your part, particularly in the early stages, might be a good idea. 'I'm always losing things, too, these days. I couldn't find my glasses this morning and they were on my head.'

Be complimentary when a person does something well. But don't be too gushing or you will risk turning compliments into meaningless 'Have a nice day' comments.

Try to get a sense of a person's attention span. But be aware when the limit is being reached. At this point it will probably be a good idea to do something different – a rest, a cup of tea or a walk.

Don't talk about yourself too much. In the past, a close relative or friend would have wanted to hear your news, but things are different now. A bit of information about what you did on holiday, perhaps accompanied by some photos is fine, but expecting a person to process a lot of facts about lengthy boat trips or ancient historic buildings might result in disengagement.

That said, in the much later stages, when a person has little expressive communication, things are different and a one-sided conversation might be appropriate. The person might simply appreciate hearing the sound of a familiar well-loved voice.

When making phone calls, you will have to make some changes. These will have to be carried out in a different way from the way they would have been in the past. The lack of cues and prompts provided by facial expressions and body language mean that this form of communication can be quite mentally taxing for a person with dementia.

Don't ever say, 'Hi, it's me' – no matter how close the relationship. Always avoid the need for mental processing by saying, 'Hi Dad, it's Rebecca.'

It is possible that the person – who might have enjoyed long chatty calls in the past – will be more comfortable with a fairly short call. You should fit in with this and keep what you say brief and to the point. Don't feel offended or rejected if the person seeks to end the call after a fairly short time – especially if they do so suddenly or without much effort to say goodbye nicely as before. They will probably have derived pleasure and reassurance from hearing a familiar voice.

Skyping

In the case of Skype calls, unless the person is in the early stages and has been familiar with Skype previously, you or someone else will almost certainly be required to assist and facilitate. One particular problem is that there can be delay on the line and so it will be especially important to allow the person extra time to respond. If the person at the other end comes in too soon or interrupts, this will be frustrating and demotivating.

Despite the comparative simplicity of operating a system that allows you to see and speak to someone on the other side of the world, there are sometimes breaks in connection and problems with sound and it would be well beyond the capabilities of most people with dementia to do battle with such issues.

Don't be put off though – this sort of modern technology adds another dimension to the kind of communication that is possible. Help the person to profit from it as long as possible.

Remember, too, though, that a person with dementia, whose daughter emigrated to Canada twenty years previously, might find it confusing to see an older version of the daughter she remembers from long ago talking on a screen.

Modern internet services like this hold out great possibilities for communication but they will not be right for everybody.

A person's ability to converse diminishes with the advance of dementia. One aspect of this is that a person might suddenly change topic midstream or terminate a conversation halfway through. This is fine. The person doubtless got something out of the conversational exchanges you did have, and a lack of a conventionally satisfactory ending is of no importance so long as the person appears untroubled.

It's all about them.

5

Language and Vocabulary

The words you choose really do matter. Your aim should be to keep the amount of mental processing expected of the person to a minimum. As always the stage the person has reached will be of great relevance – indeed in the early stages there might be little need to make any significant adjustments.

GUIDELINES FOR MAKING UNDERSTANDING EASIER

Here are some general guidelines:

Keep your words simple, everyday and concrete as far as possible. Think ahead. If you were going to say, 'Mary has just bought a really sophisticated new gadget for the kitchen that can make any kind of smoothie you fancy', think again. Say, 'Mary has a new machine . . . for making fruit juice . . . it's great', preferably at the same time as you are pointing to it. In this way you will reinforce the words with a visual cue.

Avoid abstract words like 'philosophy' or 'jealousy'.

Don't use words that could be seen as disrespectful or demeaning. Don't talk about 'feeding' the person. Say 'giving her lunch'.

Avoid complex tenses that require a greater degree of working out.

> *'It would have been nice if David had come to visit us today. I'm sure we would have had a great time.'*

Instead say:

> *'David didn't come today. Pity. Nice guy.'*

So far as possible use the present tense. If you say somebody is coming to visit the week after next, this will have little real meaning to anybody who is well into the dementia journey.

Use the active not the passive voice. Don't say, 'Jenny was taken to the day centre this morning.' This makes her sound like a parcel being delivered somewhere. Say, 'Jenny went to the day centre on the bus this morning.'

A person might be in the habit of using particular words for particular objects. Try to make yourself familiar with these words and always use them.

Do this as naturally as possible – it is a case of getting yourself into their world because this is where the best communication will take place.

If they call the family saloon a 'motor' don't refer to it as a 'car' – they will have to do a bit more work to figure out what you mean. Similarly, the person might forget the right word for an object and resort to some other term – for example a 'wiper' for a 'hanky'. If this becomes habitual then it will probably be simpler if you use this expression, too. Never appear surprised or taken aback by expressions the person uses.

Try to ensure that those people who come into contact with the person regularly are aware of words and phrases they use a lot.

If you are giving any kind of instructions or directions, be as clear as possible. Always try to avoid vagueness. If you are out walking and a person starts to veer to the right don't say, 'You're going the wrong way'– this comment does not contain much helpful information and might be taken as critical. Taking the person gently by the arm, while pointing where you are going to go, say, 'Let's go this way, left past the post office.'

Likewise, if you would like a person to pass something to you don't say, 'Could you chuck me over that thing next to the telly.' Having made sure you have their attention say, 'David . . . could you pass me the television control [pointing at the same time] . . . next to the red mug on the table beside you.'

Avoid phrases that enrich language but are not what they seem. Here are some examples along with alternative, simpler statements:

- I could murder a beer. *(I am very thirsty.)*
- I could eat a horse. *(I am very hungry.)*
- He's got skeletons in his cupboard. *(He has some secrets.)*
- He went like the clappers. *(He went very fast.)*

It might be that you know for sure that a person uses phrases like this and understands them completely – in which case fine, use them. Yet, as time goes by, a person is likely to find them increasingly confusing and even alarming and it is often safest just to avoid them.

Imagine a situation where someone suddenly coughs loudly in an unusual way – very loud and uncontrolled. If it was a friend who did not have dementia you might jokingly say you hadn't realized there was a lion in the room. If you said the same thing of a person with dementia, it is possible they would first think of some kind of literal interpretation of this and be confused, and then perhaps feel upset or confused while trying to work out what you meant. It is best to avoid such remarks altogether.

If a man is struggling to do up his belt you could take over saying, 'It's OK Dad I'll do it, you find this sort of thing tricky nowadays.' You know if you do this you will get the job done more quickly. However, the message you send to the person is confirmation that he cannot do things for himself and might thus contribute to a kind of learned helplessness. As you develop the knack of helping people with dementia you will say something like, 'Dad, doing up your belt, bit awkward . . . Can I help?' The process then becomes a kind of joint venture. It will all take slightly longer but the alternative is the risk that the person will be made to feel useless.

Sometimes, when you are talking, a person with dementia will nod in agreement as a kind of automatic social response. This does not necessarily mean that they have taken on board what you are saying. If there is any doubt, check important points: 'So Mum, we're going to the, eh . . .' said with a rising pitch at the end. The hope is you will elicit the correct answer.

ASKING QUESTIONS

As soon as you ask a person with dementia a question they immediately have to process it and then formulate a reply – which makes for a lot of mental work. As with most aspects of communication, though, it depends on the particular person and the stage they are at.

When thinking about asking a question you should first ask yourself two questions:

1. *Is it really necessary?*

2. *If so, can I get the information some other way?*

A person will realize that something is being asked of them not only from the words you use, but also from your facial expression and the rising tone of your voice at the end of the sentence. This is the point at which many will panic because by now they know that coming up with answers to any questions, however straightforward, can cause them difficulty – and this is why you have to exercise care.

As you read this you might be thinking this can't make sense. Questions are a normal, indeed essential, part of communication and it is surely unrealistic to think they can always be avoided? This is a fair general point; but you have to rethink your whole approach to communication when it comes to a person with dementia.

Here are some things to bear in mind:

Questions such as 'How are you?' are generally all right.
People will say 'Fine thanks' semi-automatically in the same

way they can count up to ten or recite old nursery rhymes. These things appear to be hard-wired and accessible for a very long time.

Start talking around a subject you wish to raise. This is a helpful approach to obtaining information – without asking a direct question. You are giving the person cues; and it is always easier for them to come up with an answer based on recognition as opposed to plucking it from the depths of their memory without any prompts beyond a bald question.

You might want to know if a particular neighbour had been in to visit recently. You could say, 'Has John been in to see you, Dad?' There is a good chance this would result in wide-eyed anxiety as the person tries to consult their memory. A better approach would be to start talking about the neighbour. 'Your neighbour John, the tall one with the grey beard, is a nice man. I like talking to him', all the time watching to see if this is sparking any recognition. You could continue by saying, 'John comes in to see you sometimes.' During this time the person has had time to tune in to the subject of John and might be enabled to say, 'John was here. We looked at some photographs.' Note that the specific day John came in is almost certainly unimportant. Exchanges like this can help to give you information without causing anxiety.

You are telling not asking – an important principle of communication with a person with dementia.

Provide prompts and cues in the question to help the person tune in. In a similar way to the previous example, don't say, 'I hear you visited the folks up north last week. How was it?' Far too vague. Having made sure you have the person's attention say something like, 'You visited David and Alison in Edinburgh, lovely big house, nice ginger cat . . .'

In the process of doing this, the hope is that the very specific information you have provided will trigger memories. Get rid of phrases like 'last week' – largely meaningless to a person with dementia beyond the early stages; they are recognizable words yes, but working out what they mean in the context of a specific question is likely to be beyond them and you have to ask yourself the question, does it matter if it was last week or the week before? Indeed, a person might home in on a phrase like this, thinking they should know whether it was last week or the week before, and then become bogged down with this detail rather than focus on the meat of the question.

And don't look for social niceties; don't expect the person to wait until you have finished speaking before taking their turn.

Assuming they start speaking – whenever this occurs – that is the time for you to stop and then to tune into what they are saying and give them suitable prompts to continue and, you hope, provide the information you are after.

Now some people might take the view that this is all too much bother, and anyway the person does not seem very interested in chatting. Although there might be times when a person is tired or affected by their medication and therefore not keen on talking, such occasions will generally be the exception. Most people want social exchanges – wouldn't you? But their condition can make it harder and they need your help.

Avoid open questions

Don't say, 'What would you like to drink?' This opens up the whole world of beverages of every description – a huge amount to consider and process. Having got the person's attention, say, 'Gran . . . tea or coffee?' The choices offered should of course be based on the time of day and your prior knowledge of the person's preferences. Similarly, when helping a person to get dressed you could simply say 'What do you want to wear today?' Alternatively you could go to the other extreme: present them with some clothes and say, 'Here's what you're wearing today.' A better idea would be to show them a few items of clothing and ask which one they would prefer.

You are respecting the person's right to make a choice but not giving them too much to think about.

In the early stages it will almost certainly not be necessary to simplify things to this extent. Much later on, even such basic choices will be unrealistic. You will make decisions based on your knowledge of their preferences.

Avoid hypothetical questions

'What would you do if you won the lottery?' Like open questions, hypothetical questions involve a great deal of mental processing, in particular consulting the imagination.

Avoid asking for specific detailed information about events in the recent past

Here are two examples:

1. 'Was Joan here last Thursday?' Most people would find it hard to say what they were doing last Thursday; for people

with dementia it will be next to impossible. It might well also serve to remind them of their problems and be demoralizing.

2. 'What did you have for breakfast?' This, too, involves accessing the most recent memory, the worst affected area – and does it really matter? If for some reason it does, you could start talking about breakfast topics as in the earlier example of the neighbour John in the hope this will take you to what you want to know.

Make use of prompts and cues

If you say, 'Dad . . . would you like to sit down?' pat the chair at the same time, or point to it. Wherever possible try to back up words with actions, mime, gesture, and so on.

You have to get into a mind-set that looks at situations from the point of the view of the person with dementia. What will make comprehension of spoken words easiest for them?

A lot of people have got the message from the media that if they give people with dementia quiz-type tests or exercises – 'What is the capital of Egypt?' or 'What do the letters MP stand for?' – or word games, this might somehow help to delay the progress of their condition by keeping their brains active. There might be an element of truth in this. In addition, if a person, prior to the onset of their condition, engaged in a lot of mentally demanding activities then this might help them to be better able to devise strategies to counteract their failing powers for longer than people who did not do such activities. There are, however, differing views on this subject.

However, if you compel a person with dementia to engage in such activities as some kind of brain-stretching therapy, there is a considerable risk that you will simply make them feel anxious and uneasy.

They might well think something along the lines of, 'I understand the question. I should know the answer but I just can't think of it. What an idiot I am. Why are they putting me through this?' Would you want a relative or friend to feel like this?

Having said all this, there are people, probably in the earlier stages, who are keen to get involved in such exercises. Fine – so long as you are sure this genuinely reflects their wishes.

One strategy is to ask questions to which the answer is yes or no. This can work for particular situations, 'Would you like a cup of tea?', 'Are you cold?', or 'Are you tired?' However, such questions have clear limitations for developing any kind of conversation.

CONVERSATION ISSUES

Any kind of conversational exchange with a person with dementia can present problems not usually encountered when you are talking with a person who does not have dementia. Here are a few examples, together with possible ways of dealing with them.

If a person loses the thread of what they were saying you could:

1. As naturally as possible give a brief summary of what they were saying: 'You were telling me about your time in Malta during the war . . .'

2. Ask a question which is framed as a statement and which acts as a prompt: 'Something to do with Mary.'

3. Encourage them to say anything at all on the subject they were talking about or to try to say it in another way in the hope that this gets round the blockage. You are not saying it for them but simply helping them to say it. It might be that they are just collecting their thoughts and a simple prompt of this sort will get them back on track. It might also be the case that something more compelling has come into their mind, in which case they should be encouraged to move on to that.

Be flexible. Don't try to bring a person back to a subject they have chosen to move on from.

If it becomes clear that a person has lost the thread of a particular subject you can gently move things on by taking the lead and saying for instance, 'Now let's talk about . . .'

If a person is talking about something quite successfully but struggles to find a particular word and you think you know what it is, try not to say it for them. If you think the word is 'wheelchair', you could discreetly say the first sound of the word with a look somewhere between questioning and encouragement, 'Whee . . .' A prompt of this sort might well be enough to give them the word.

You could also – if you are sure you know the word the person is looking for – pretend that you, too, have the word on the tip of your tongue and enter a kind of joint search to find it, in the course of which you provide clues or cues which enable them to get the answer: 'Oh I know what you mean, what is it now? It's that fruit, the yellow one you peel . . .'

Be prepared to be flexible and think outside the box; as an alternative to saying something, mime it or ask the person to draw it or even write it down or draw a picture of it – whatever feels right.

Rather than engaging in the mild subterfuge of the foregoing strategies you could simply say something like, 'You seem to be having a problem here, is it OK if I help?' and then deploy whatever strategy seems right.

You might also judge there to be times when it is best just to say the word yourself in order to move things on, but wherever possible try to help the person to produce it themselves.

As you can doubtless imagine, all of this will involve trial and error.

If a person says something that is factually wrong the right thing to do in most cases is not to correct them. There is no point. You will simply remind the person that their memory is not working efficiently. If they saw the doctor two weeks ago but say it was yesterday, then that is their reality and you should not presume to change it. Indeed if you do, it is tantamount to telling them they are lying – because when they say it they believe it to be true.

Under no circumstances should you ever get into any kind of argument or heated debate over some factual details. This would be completely pointless and could cause a lot of anxiety and upset.

Bear in mind also that, there is a very good chance that if you do contradict the person or try to insist on getting them to accept the truth, they might appear to take them in momentarily but then forget them soon afterwards – and so nothing positive will have been achieved.

If, however, you do judge it would be worthwhile to correct a detail – and this should be the exception – there are ways in which this might be achieved without causing upset.

If a person said they saw Helen when in fact it was Maria you could say, 'Sorry, I missed that, did you say you saw Maria?' The chances are the person will pause momentarily and say 'Oh yes, Maria . . .' and move on. Don't say, 'Helen? Don't think so, must have been someone else – surely it was Maria?'

Similarly, if a person looked out of the window at heavy rain and said, 'It's really snowing heavily', you could reply to them and say matter-of-factly, 'Yes it really is raining a lot.' The person might well pick up on your correction but without feeling they have been put down in any way.

This kind of correction will be of greater importance if, say, a person has confused the names of two grandchildren – you have to think of the feelings of the children too. That said, children are often understanding and accepting if it is simply explained to them that Grandpa has a problem with his memory and gets mixed up sometimes.

In similar vein, when, as is very common, a person uses empty words such as 'thingummy' you can supply the missing detail in your reply. For instance a person might say, 'David got a new thingummy', to which you could say, 'Oh yes I saw David's new camera, very good.' This is not a question of trying to teach the person new language but simply helping to fill out or enrich a conversation they want to initiate or take part in.

As the condition progresses, a person with dementia will lose what might be called the social graces of language. You will ask how they are but they might well not reciprocate. This can be particularly hard to come to terms with if the person has always been interested in others and concerned about their feelings. They might interrupt you or talk across you, in which case, as a general rule, you should go with what they want to talk about; don't tell them to wait until you have finished what you are saying. Their behaviour is a result of their condition. Don't be offended – not even if at some point the person falls asleep.

Be pleased that you have spent a bit of time with them and, you hope, given them some moments of pleasure.

A little bit of empathy can sometimes help to reduce the kind of anxiety a person feels when they can't find a word or lose their thread. You could say, 'Sometimes it is hard to find the right word' or 'I find the older I get, the more often I forget things.'

These remarks might qualify as minor white lies (then again, maybe not) but that is unimportant if they serve to make the person feel less stressed and conversation easier.

Any such strategies would of course be beyond the capability of a person with dementia. Don't expect any empathy from them for any stress or difficulties you experience when you are with them.

If a person says something you find it hard to make sense of, you might ask them to repeat it or try to talk around it once or twice but you don't want to be doing this repeatedly. In general, you should try to avoid saying you follow what a person says when you don't. However, there will probably be times when this is unavoidable – the least worst option. If this happens try to be a bit vague – a nod, a smile, a general acceptance. Say something generally supportive – 'It's nice talking to you.' Do not look blank or uncomprehending.

If there are particular words which recur, and which do not make sense to you, particularly in the later stages, you could discreetly note them down and then do a bit of detective work with relatives and friends to see if any light can be thrown on them from the person's past. Thereafter you could try to get back on to that topic in the hope of enabling the person to say more.

If a person appears to use words or phrases in a strange way, don't dismiss them. It might be that they contain meaning that is just not immediately apparent. People with dementia might well find themselves wanting to express something but be unable to produce the words they would have used in the past, the ones that would make most sense to you.

If a person said, 'My brain got pulled out and burnt to hell' or 'I'm dragging this stone up the hill', you might think they were making no sense. However, it might be a case of a person expressing frustration at feelings of hopelessness or their inability to speak, think or reason as they did in the past – in the best way that their current mental processes will permit them. In fact it is not too hard to see meaning in these particular phrases – it will not always be so easy.

It can be unsettling when a person talks about things from the past as if they are in the present.

However, you have to remember that for them this is the reality they are experiencing at that moment and you should not seek to take them out of their world and into the real here and now version.

They are not being forgetful in a normal way; as a result of their condition they think what they say is true. Perhaps the next day they will not talk in this way. Thoughts and words can swim up to the surface in unpredictable ways.

As a general point too, remember that any conversational exchange that works is giving something of value to a person – no matter how short. But don't be surprised if the next time you see them they have forgotten all about it. This is normal. Don't take offence.

Conversing in general company

If you are with a person with dementia and other people who do not have dementia, it is only too easy to get into a conversation with those who don't. If we are honest, it is often a relief to be talking in a normal way again; indeed you can almost forget that the person is there – and they will probably not try to join the conversation.

However, you might say things which could alarm the person with dementia. You might say for instance, talking about some person at your workplace, 'I saw John yesterday; he's so pompous, I find him very hard going, not a nice guy at all.' You would say this in all innocence at your usual conversational speed. Unfortunately the person with dementia might just pick up a few words and wonder whether you were talking about them; unable to express their concern, they might just feel uncomfortable.

In general, if you wish to have an easy-going chat with a friend, try to do so when you are on your own with them.

If you wish to discuss some important matter of relevance to a person with dementia with relatives or friends, it is generally better not to do so in the presence of the person. The matters raised and the language caused might cause alarm or confusion. If there is something that does need to be communicated to the person with dementia following on from your discussion, tell them later.

It is sad in some ways that language has to be simplified and impoverished, but it is in the best interests of the person with dementia. But do not go to extremes; develop a knack for striking a balance. If you simplify things too much too soon, this might come over as patronizing. In the later stages, however, your language and vocabulary will have to be considerably stripped down if the best possible communication is to be achieved.

Another element of acquiring the skill of carrying out the most helpful and appropriate behaviour is self-monitoring. If you say something and immediately think it worked well, or was a mistake, learn from this; add it to your personal collection of what does and doesn't work.

BEGINNINGS AND ENDINGS

If you call in on a friend or relative who does not have dementia you might well burst into the room, ask questions, get into a chat about what has been happening, all at high speed, with the television on in the corner of the room. Do that to a person with dementia and you are all but guaranteed to raise their stress and confusion levels as they desperately try to make sense of what is going on.

How you start and finish any kind of visit or contact requires a little forethought. It is all part of the knack of communicating well.

As a general principle, do not initiate any conversation with a person until you have made sure they know who you are and are tuned into the fact that you are going to say something. An exchange with an old friend called Derek might go something like this, just after you have entered the room:

YOU: 'Derek.'

PAUSE. Make eye contact, touch Derek's arm, shake his hand, smile – whatever feels most natural and appropriate.

YOU: 'Hi, it's Martha.' (Even if you have known the person for a long time, it is a good idea to matter-of-factly state your name. The last thing you want is to put the person in a position of having to test their memory to get your name.)

PAUSE. Look for signs of recognition.

YOU: 'Good to see you. How are you Derek?'

If you live with the person you will get to know their routines. The chances are that as time goes on, the person will not get going quickly in the morning. Accordingly, greetings at this time should be similar each day and should not include information about what will be happening during the day. Save that for when the person is up and about and has had breakfast and any medication.

Physical contact can be helpful when establishing initial contact. A prolonged handshake, good but not overly intense eye contact, and perhaps an arm round the shoulder or a hug. Do not, however, assume that everybody will welcome this. Most will, but there are gender, cultural and religious issues to be taken into account. Just try to be as sensitive and responsive to the person as possible. Base what you do on your knowledge of the person or that of someone who knows them better than you.

Initial contact with professionals. Contact with doctors, lawyers, social workers or visitors who are not well known to the person is one particularly important function you will have to carry out as the person's advocate.

You will almost certainly be doing the introductions and making the opening statements. This is an area of communication the person would, of course, have taken care of themselves in the past.

In the case of meetings with health or other professionals, you should make sure you are as well informed as possible in advance. This will involve clarifying the person's view of their symptoms and wishes. It will probably be a good idea to make some notes. Once a meeting has started, your role will be as a kind of go-between. You will help to explain the person's problem, encourage the person to speak and express their views, and then make sure they understand what is said in response. It might be that some of the explaining will have to be done back home.

As part of any initial contact, try to assess a person's demeanour. What messages is the person with dementia giving you? Do they look tired? Are their facial muscles tensed up? Do they seem quite bright? Answers to these questions will help guide you in what it might be appropriate to do with them during your visit. For instance, if the person seems tired or lacking energy it might be best to sit and talk or watch something on television. If they appear more energetic then a walk in the park might be more appropriate.

If you leave the room for a significant amount of time remember that the person, when their condition is more advanced, might well forget that you had been there. Don't burst into the room and expect to continue where you left off. A brief re-introduction will be helpful to resume contact. You might simply tell the person that you had been in the garden – or wherever. Your aim is to avoid doing anything that takes them by surprise.

Remember that the person will probably not have been thinking about your departure. When the time approaches for you to leave, it might come as something of an unwelcome surprise. Accordingly, when the time comes it will be a good idea to prepare the person. Mention in passing that you will have to be getting back soon some time before you actually leave. Do this again as the time gets nearer. You could perhaps pick up your coat and place it across your knee as you say it.

Try to end on a positive note. Thank the person. Give the impression that you have had a pleasant time and that the person made a valuable contribution to this. As with the start of the visit, some warm physical contact will almost certainly be a good idea. All of these things communicate a message of valuing the person. You might well say that you will see them again soon and be quite definite on the point.

Yet there is little point in saying that you will call again a week on Thursday at three – it is highly unlikely that this will be meaningful and it might just cause anxiety as the person tries to work out what that means exactly or memorize it. If you do know the specific date you will return you could, however, note it in the person's diary and show them the entry.

Arrange things so that someone else is with the person when you leave. Doing so has the effect of softening the blow, but of course it will not always be possible.

CHOOSING TOPICS TO TALK ABOUT

It is quite a good idea on meeting a person with dementia to try and establish if they do actually want to talk. There will be times when they are tired or affected by drugs and will be happier just to sit with you and appreciate your company with only a few comments here and there. This is fine. The fact that you are there is giving them companionship and communicating an unstated message of friendship and support. You should never cajole a person into talking or taking part in conversation or an activity if it is clear they don't want to. There will be other opportunities.

It is more likely, however, that the person will be keen to talk. Your aim should be to find subjects that will make conversation as easy as possible – and those which will work best will be the ones that reflect the person's own view of things.

◆ A good starting point is to try to home in on what the person is doing when you meet them. Perhaps they're watching television or doing something in the garden or patting a dog. Whatever the action, this will be the most recent thing in their thoughts and you should try to stay with that, develop and expand it any way you can.

◆ If you are a friend who visits from time to time, ask close relatives in advance what kinds of topics the person is or has been interested in – the war, work, holidays, hobbies, pets – and use these as starting points.

◆ Old photographs and other items from the past can be very helpful triggers – this subject is dealt with in Chapter 9.

◆ Men and women are often interested in talking about different things. One way into conversation might be for a woman to say to another woman, 'I wasn't sure what to wear today. Do you think this top goes with this skirt?' whilst doing a twirl. The gesture and a questioning tone of voice will make it easier for the person to tune in. In this way you are the one raising the subject but you are also getting into the person's views right away.

◆ You could use the same approach – for men and women – with a whole range of subjects, from cookery and cars to holidays and pets. The use of photographs or brochures in association with what you are saying will always be helpful.

◆ In the advanced stages a person might come out with words or actions that do not appear to make any sense. One technique that will generate some kind of conversational exchange and help the person to express themselves is simply to repeat the words or actions back to them, perhaps also making up phrases which feature the words, in the hope that this will make it easier for the person to expand upon what they were saying.

◆ If you have the kind of personality that likes playing imaginative games, you can find that a simple exchange like this can lead to a reaction from the person with dementia, more words and eventually some kind of communication: a kind of verbal table tennis.

◆ Bear in mind that like most people, a person with dementia will have some painful memories in their past. Close family members will be aware of such things but if you don't know the person too well, make sure you enquire in advance about any areas that are best avoided.

6

Non-Verbal Communication

Communication is about much more than mere words. Non-verbal communication accounts for a large part of the way human beings send messages to one another. Estimates vary but many put the figure at about 90 per cent. Yes, 90 per cent. According to this way of thinking, communication can roughly be split up as follows:

◆ Words: 10 per cent

◆ Tone, volume, speed and pitch of voice, etc.: 40 per cent

◆ Gesture, posture, facial expressions, body language, etc.: 50 per cent

These figures are not exact but nonetheless it is strikingly clear that the stuff other than words constitutes a major element of communication.

Non-verbal communication can take a great many forms, some of them operating at a sub-conscious level. It helps to clarify, reinforce and give meaning to the words you say. As dementia progresses, non-verbal communication will become increasingly important as words become more difficult to process. Indeed in some situations you might not use words at all.

Most of us use non-verbal communication, such as hand movements, automatically, without any planning or forethought. Sometimes, though, we will be more deliberate. A defence lawyer might lower his voice dramatically before raising it again suddenly and then saying forcefully, 'Ladies and gentlemen of the jury, I urge you to acquit an innocent man!' He might well reinforce his words by staring at the jury members whilst leaning towards them and then remaining silent for a while and gently nodding his head in order to let the message contained in his words sink in.

You only have to think about the facial expressions and vocal acrobatics of comedians such as John Cleese, Billy Connolly, Lenny Henry and Michael McIntyre – and countless others – to realize just how much expressive value is added to the comparatively small number of words they actually use to tell a story. When you add in the meaningful pauses, the physical gestures, the sudden movements, the changes of pace, it is not hard to see that the apparently surprising figure of around 90 per cent is probably not far off the mark.

There are an infinite number of examples of non-verbal communication of particular relevance to people with dementia – as well of course to people who interact with them. The ones covered in this chapter will give you an idea of some of them. You will come across others in the course of looking after a person that will be unique to them.

SMILING

This is one of the commonest and most important forms of non-verbal communication. People with dementia often have feelings of anxiety, alarm or fear for any number of reasons, and a smile will help to provide reassurance. You should get into the habit of smiling quite a lot, particularly when you think the person is experiencing such negative feelings. A word of warning, however – don't overdo it. If you do, there is a risk that you will come over as insincere. As a very rough guide, think about how much you smile normally and increase it by about 20 per cent.

Bear in mind also the other side of the coin: you should try to avoid drifting off into very serious or glum looks or grimaces – the person might read negative implications into them and feel concerned.

The way you communicate has considerable power to influence your relationships in a way that is different from the everyday communication you have with people who do not have dementia; and it requires more effort and concentration.

PITCH AND TONE OF VOICE

The way you say things does a lot to emphasize or add meaning to what you vocalize. If you say it loudly, this could indicate irritation, emphasis or merely the fact that you think somebody might have difficulty hearing what you say. If you say the same thing gently, this could express sensitivity, sympathy or could indicate a concern not to disturb another nearby person.

If you raise the pitch of your voice at the end of a sentence, this indicates a question. If you lower the pitch at the end of a sentence, it generally indicates that you have finished what you want to say. Try to be aware of the likely impact of such variations on the person you are talking to – monitor their reactions and make appropriate adjustments.

As part of recasting the way you communicate with a person, you should consider exaggerating these things a bit in order to add emphasis to what you are saying – but the point about not overdoing it applies. Remember also that if a person does not respond or does not appear particularly interested in what you say they are not being thoughtless or unkind. You should not take this as personally as you might well do if you were talking to a person who did not have dementia.

CRYING

Sometimes people with dementia can become emotional very quickly and you might be unaware of the cause. Crying gives a very strong message that the person is experiencing a powerful emotion and you should stop whatever you are doing, give the person your attention and use good communication skills to try to ascertain the cause. Do not try to stop the person crying – it can be a valuable form of expression that can provide relief – but do offer comfort and make it clear that you want to help.

AGITATED ACTIONS

If a person starts fussing with an article of clothing, a shoe or their belt, or a part of their body, or is clearly agitated and restless – but does not express any concerns verbally – it is up to you to try to find out what message they are sending and then to address the problem. For example, if you notice a woman starting to pull up her skirt as she sits down in a chair, this is likely to be a sign that she needs to go to the toilet.

Similarly, if a person physically pushes you away, or holds up a flat hand towards you, this is a dramatic non-verbal way of telling you that something has upset them in some way and you should respond to this as you would if a person started crying. Try to lower the emotional temperature as the first step towards understanding and addressing the problem.

SWEATING AND MUSCLE TENSION

If a person is sweating for no immediately apparent reason, this is telling you something. It might be a sign of anxiety or illness or quite simply that the heating is set too high. Once more, assuming the person does not provide you with a clear spoken explanation, your investigative skills will be called upon to locate the cause.

In addition, be aware of any muscle tension in a person's face, which might betray feelings of pain or discomfort – even though they might, in answer to questions, say that everything is all right.

POSTURE, BODY LANGUAGE AND PERSONAL SPACE

If a person is slumped in a chair, a negative message is being given off; the person looks dejected and helpless and for some visitors, less approachable – the last thing you want when trying to encourage people to engage with the person. Also, as mentioned previously, poor posture can make a person's voice production weaker.

Your own posture can also be an important element of communication. Your aim is to appear non-threatening and available for the person with dementia. You want to give the impression that they are the focus of your attention. Try to appear relaxed and open – whether sitting or standing. Don't have your arms folded around your middle.

Try to be aware of how physically close a person wants you to be. This might well not be an issue with relatives or very good friends. However, with less well-known people a person might feel uncomfortable or in some way intimidated if a visitor gets too close. They might not express this in words and so you have to watch for any non-verbal signs such as turning their face away.

AROMAS

If it is getting close to lunchtime and some aromas drift through from the kitchen, you could exploit this. Stop what you are doing, ensure you have the person's attention, breathe in the aroma in a slightly exaggerated way, give a look of pleasure and then say, 'Lunch time', while gesturing towards the kitchen or dining room. This will act as a prompt and help to stimulate the person's appetite. Likewise, the noise of plates and cutlery being put on the table could be used to indicate that it is time to get ready for a meal.

Aromas do have their limitations, though. In the earlier stages such strategies will not be necessary. In the later stages it is less likely that the person will be so responsive to these kinds of prompts – more directive action, such as clear statements and gestures, will probably be required.

MUSIC

Music can play an important role in the life of a person with dementia in a number of ways. It can provide pleasing, evocative and colourful sounds in the way that it can for everybody. It can do more than this, however; research has shown that music can reduce levels of stress and agitation and soothe feelings of aggression or paranoia in people with dementia; and what's more there are no side effects. One writer has described music as a non-pharmacological sedative. There is also some research which suggests that music can help to unlock memories from the past and bring them to the surface.

However, there are a number of important points to make:

◆ It might seem an obvious point, but you should play music that is familiar to and liked by the person, always bearing in mind that a person's tastes can change over time.

◆ As a general rule, up-to-the-minute modern music should be avoided. Notably, radio stations playing pop music often have a great deal of fast talk which a person with dementia will not follow. It is unlikely that any of this will be pleasing to their ear, though as with so much else, they might not find it easy to express this.

◆ For as long as possible, try to enable the person to play music without your assistance. Have a CD player in an obvious place with a set of simple instructions on the wall next to it – though assuming the person has been in the habit of playing CDs in the past, such instructions will probably not be necessary for quite a time. There will eventually come a stage when you will be the one who initiates the playing of music.

◆ Some studies have shown that classical music tends to be more relaxing for people with dementia and that it can have the effect of reducing agitation and stress levels. Accordingly, if for any reason it is not possible to play familiar, well-loved music, then classical will probably create a more pleasant musical environment than pop – but it really depends on the individual.

◆ Remember, too, that some pieces of music can be associated with unhappy events from the past – try as far as possible to be aware of such music and avoid it.

◆ Consider putting together personalized compilations of music you know the person likes.

◆ There are websites that enable you to play virtually unlimited amounts of music from particular artists or genres.

SENDING OUT NEGATIVE MESSAGES

Just because a person has dementia it does not mean that they do not pick up negative messages you might give out non-verbally. If you have been asked the same question many times it is very hard not to feel exasperated and to show this by, for example, raising your eyes to heaven whilst at the same time saying, 'It's OK.' Although it is often not possible to know for certain what is in the mind of a person with dementia, they might well be upset at the thought that they were the cause of your negative feelings. Some experts think that people with dementia can have a heightened ability to read non-verbal signs.

It is a counsel of perfection which you will not always achieve, but resolute and good-natured patience will help to keep a person with dementia on an even keel.

If there are times when you find things particularly tough, it is probably a good idea to get away from the situation altogether for a while. Go for a walk, meditate, go to the shops, offload to a friend – break the cycle. It is not realistic to expect a person with dementia to understand your feelings, make allowances and adjust their behaviour.

USING GESTURES, MIME, SIGN LANGUAGE AND FACIAL EXPRESSION

If you want to offer a person a cup of tea you could:

Walk up to them and say in a flat voice, 'Would you like a cup of tea?' In the middle to later stages even a simple question like this could be difficult for the person to process. To make it easier for them, as you say the words:

◆ Widen your eyes/raise your eyebrows.
◆ Raise the pitch of your voice at the end of the question.
◆ Hold your two index fingers in the shape of a T.
◆ Slightly tilt your head to one side.

As with verbal communication, always allow a person time to respond – non-verbal gestures also require a degree of mental processing.

There are countless situations where gestures will back up words; you should develop your own basic sign language to make communication easier.

Here are a few more examples:

◆ A thumbs-up or -down sign for good or bad.

◆ Touching a plate and suddenly withdrawing your hand to indicate it is hot.

◆ Putting your hands together and placing them against the side of your leaning head to indicate time for bed.

◆ Miming brushing teeth prior to going into bathroom.

◆ Putting your hands round your middle and saying, 'Brrrrr' to indicate that it is cold and that a coat will be necessary for going outside.

The possibilities are endless. You will doubtless use some of these gestures when talking to people who do not have dementia – they are everyday supplements to words. However, in the case of a person with dementia their use should be more targeted and deliberate.

It is not a bad idea to introduce a few gestures in the early to middle stages, before they are really necessary. The hope is that they will become familiar and might help to facilitate communication later on when a person's ability to understand words has diminished further and gesture has become a key element of communication.

Please note, by the way, that none of this amounts to treating the person like a child – it is a case of finding practical ways of dealing with the communication problems caused by dementia.

In the last stages, when a person has had dementia for many years, it can be hard to believe they are capable of much meaningful communication at all. Whilst it is true that overt conventional communication might have almost disappeared, this does not mean it has been entirely extinguished. It will, however, entail a certain amount of guesswork and following of hunches.

In addition, it is important to make certain assumptions, principally that:

The person is still there.
The person would like to have company.
The person would like to have some kind of communicative stimulation.

This does not always happen and people who live long enough to reach the most advanced stages of dementia are sometimes left alone for lengthy periods of time because the people charged with their care assume that because they have lost the ability to express wishes, they don't have any.

There are many professionals who believe that, with the right approach, it is possible to have some level of communication with people almost to the end of life – one-sided conversations, music and stroking of their hands, for example. Some compare communicating with a person in the last stages of dementia with communicating with someone in a coma. It is a large subject, which can only be touched on in this book; however, one important point is that you should look for communication by the person in the smallest of gestures:

◆ Small movements of the eyes.
◆ Slight movements of the head.
◆ Slight facial expressions of pain or relief.

As has been mentioned before, looking after a person with dementia can involve a certain amount of detective work and this is particularly true in the final stages. If you put a light on, play a piece of music or present a drink, watch for any gestures at all and try to interpret them and respond accordingly. For instance, if you turn on a light and it seems that the person reacts with a slightly pained expression, turn the light off. As basic as that.

CLOTHES

Clothes can say a lot about a person. Some people are more interested than others in what they wear, but everybody makes choices that are indicative of their personal identity. This is true for people with dementia too, but they will find it harder to exercise choice and make sure they are wearing what they want on a particular day or for a particular occasion. They will need help – although as time goes on the whole experience will be very different from the past, which included carefree shopping expeditions and lots of choice.

Your aim should be to help the person wear the kind of clothes they prefer and which say something about who they are.

Clothes can also be triggers for conversation, for instance you could comment on the length of skirts in the past or how shoes used to be all about practicality as opposed to fashion.

A person may well want to wear familiar clothes, which will help to maintain continuity in their lives. Accordingly, clothes you might think are a bit faded and past their best will still be chosen – perhaps some fixing and mending will be required. Try to involve the person in buying new clothes when the need arises.

Whatever clothes are chosen they should be clean, free of marks, and well ironed where appropriate. If this does not happen the message will be given that the person is not worth the trouble it takes to attend to such things. Visitors will doubtless get a similar message.

Clothes can act as prompts in various situations. For instance, as it gets late, you could discreetly produce the person's dressing gown and slippers and place them within their sight. This will communicate the message that it will soon be time for bed and might make the whole process easier when you come to say the words. Similarly, if you are planning an outing, you could produce an overcoat, gloves or umbrella shortly beforehand.

Bear in mind also that whenever you are planning to move from one activity or place to another, this should happen gradually so that the person has a chance to adjust to the new situation. Never start putting on a person's coat as you hurriedly tell them that it is time to go out – that could cause confusion and alarm. Think ahead.

Most of the points that apply to clothes also apply to hair styling. In the later stages you might be tempted to go for something purely practical, but it really is such an important part of a person's image – especially a woman's – that you should try to maintain some version of their preferred hair style for as long as possible.

PHYSICAL CONTACT

There appears to be universal agreement that physical contact with a person with dementia can communicate a wide variety of desirable positive messages. However, take care. There will be some people who will feel uneasy about physical contact. There could be many reasons for this: upbringing, gender issues, a trauma from the past, cultural or religious strictures and so on. Obviously, if the person in question is a close friend or relative you will have a very good idea of their feelings on the subject, but bear in mind that these feelings could change under the influence of their condition.

You should monitor, and be sensitive to, the responses of a person. You will soon get an understanding of what they are comfortable with.

But none of this alters the general principle that physical contact can be a very good thing indeed. People with dementia – like everybody else – want some physical contact, but their condition makes it harder for them to express such desires, which can often go unmet. Some researchers believe that the need and desire for physical contact increases with age.

It might be that you are not the sort of person who particularly likes or feels comfortable with physical contact – in which case you should try to have as much contact as you do feel comfortable with. You might be pleasantly surprised at how easy and pleasurable it is for you, too, once you have taken the plunge and overcome your inhibitions.

As a matter of interest, there is research which has found that in general women are happier about giving and receiving physical contact than men.

As mentioned earlier, it can be very helpful, in order to be sure you have a person's attention, to touch them gently on the arm. Hugs, handshakes, arms around shoulders and pats on the back can also transmit positive messages and might also be soothing if a person is agitated for any reason.

Do bear in mind, though, that when you are about to make physical contact with a person you should not come at them suddenly, without warning or from behind. Make sure the person has seen you and had a chance to register your identity, and that physical contact is imminent. Likewise, if you are going to go out somewhere with the person, do not suddenly take their wrist and pull them towards the door. This might spark off childhood memories of being punished by teachers or parents and cause alarm.

A slow and ever so slightly tentative approach is generally best.

Physical contact also holds some more intimate communicative possibilities.

Holding hands – if you have any doubt about the powerful messages this simple action can send, just think back to when you held hands with your first boyfriend or girlfriend.

A back, hand or foot massage – particularly with pleasantly scented oils or cream – can provide pleasure and relaxation whilst at the same time sending out a deep message of closeness. The same applies to washing and brushing hair. These are forms of communication that require few words, which bypass the complications of conversation and which are therefore not in any way challenging for the receiver. That said, the effect might also be to make one-to-one conversation flow more easily and naturally.

If you treat this kind of contact as a sort of therapeutic treatment, it could help to dispel any feelings of awkwardness about such close physical contact on either side. You might find that a brief hand massage prior to an event that you know might be stressful – a trip to the doctor, for instance – will help to calm the person.

A wet shave for a man is another sensory experience you might include. It can feel strange to do this for, say, a father or uncle, but just think of the pleasure you will give and the message you will send to the person: you are saying, without words, that you care about them. Such an experience might also help to generate some good quality spoken conversation.

Sexual union can provide great comfort and send positive messages even when a person's ability to express love in other ways is becoming limited. If you are in a relationship with a person with dementia and sex has been a part of your relationship, in principle there is no reason why this should not continue for a reasonable length of time.

There can, however, be difficulties associated with sexual relations, which are addressed in Chapter 10.

Touch can be particularly important in the later stages of life because other channels of communication are no longer available. Although you cannot always be absolutely sure, it is highly likely that physical contact such as holding and stroking a person's hand or head will transmit a message of reassurance and provide comfort.

In the very last stages, if a person reaches the stage of being bedbound with very little obvious communicative ability, there are people who believe the best way of finally communicating feelings of human warmth and love is to get into bed beside the person and hold them. It is similar to what you would do with a newborn baby and could be seen as life coming full circle.

7

Activities, Dementia and Communication

ACTIVITIES ARE ALL ABOUT COMMUNICATION

Activities involve two or more people doing things together and
this means talking, listening, observing, physically responding,
smiling, touching – as well as carrying out particular sets of
actions. People with dementia, like most other people, value and
benefit from the stimulation provided by all sorts of activities
and – even though they might not express it in words – they will
also appreciate the underlying message that somebody regards
it as worthwhile to invest time and energy in facilitating and
participating in stimulating pastimes with them.

Activities can also enable people with dementia to express
themselves or communicate things that with words would be
difficult; it is possible too that the stimulation provided will
enhance and sharpen the abilities which they retain. Some
researchers have found that well-chosen, absorbing activities
can lead to an increase in verbal fluency and a reduction in
word-finding difficulties.

In addition, activities can provide an excellent change of pace
from the many repetitive tasks that are a part of daily life.

The positive message for the person is that although life does involve a lot of mundane repetition, there are pleasant things to look forward to, that life can still be good. This can be highly motivational.

Engaging in activities to the best of their current ability also allows a person with dementia to send a message to the world that they can still do things and should not be written off.

However, as with so much else, the person will require your help – more or less depending on the stage their condition has reached. You also have to make allowances for any physical conditions such as arthritis, which render some activities difficult or unrealistic. You will need to be the main initiator and will have to come up with adaptations so that activities are definitely within the capabilities of the person. Your aim should be to come up with pleasant activities, which are not particularly demanding.

And as with communication generally, you must not assume that the old ways will work.

Here are a number of important points to bear in mind:

You should not find yourself providing detailed explanations that you need the person to take on board. Whatever the activity, try to avoid new learning other than simple physical actions, so that the person can copy them. Learning straightforward new activities in this way will probably be realistic in the early to middle stages but should be discontinued or avoided if you see anxious looks on the person's face.

Ideally look for activities, or variations of activities, which are already familiar. People are more likely to remember the steps involved in doing things they did a lot in the past, hobbies or other activities which were perhaps associated with jobs, such as cooking or drawing patterns.

It is generally not a good idea to say to a person something like, 'What would you like to do?' Unless a person is in the earlier stages, there will be too much to think about in response to an open question of this sort. You should suggest a small number of activities, based on your knowledge of their preferences, and let them choose. In the later stages, it might be more appropriate to decide on an activity you are confident the person likes and then to start doing it.

Make sure that you plan ahead and that the time is suitable for the person and you have prepared any materials in advance. The idea is that as you start doing the activity, the person will observe, access some memories of the activity, and then simply start joining in or taking over completely – something you should make as easy as possible with encouraging actions and gestures. It might be that further on you will need to be quite directive by, for example, putting a potato peeler in the person's hand.

Aim to make the person feel that the two of you are doing something together. You will of course have to initiate and be in charge much of the time, but the person should feel they have some say in how the activity is conducted.

One of the most important things to remember at all times is this: what matters is the taking part, not the final outcome.

The person might not finish the job, might lose interest after a short time or might not do an activity very well. None of this matters one little bit when set against the potential pleasure and stimulation they will get from participating. Resist any temptation to compel a person to finish something if it is clear they have lost interest. Resist, too, any personal feelings of disappointment you might have that something was not completed. It is not about you; value whatever it is the person has succeeded in doing.

Always express some admiration for what has been achieved. Do this no matter how well or badly an activity goes – without being overly gushing.

When a particular activity goes well be sure to tell other people. By telling those who spend time with the person, you can contribute to the development of a repertoire of activities the person likes.

Do not come up with things that are likely to be at or beyond the limit of a person's capabilities. Their mental capacity is impaired and will deteriorate further as time goes by. You are unlikely to achieve much by trying to stretch them. Indeed if you give them things to do that are beyond their capability, you will risk causing agitation, and remind them of what they have lost. Aim for their current level of ability or a little bit less. It is not an exact science but the more you try things out, the more you will get the knack. But do not give a person in the early stages something to do that is far too easy for them.

Get the views of other people. If you are in any doubt about the suitability of a particular activity, don't hesitate to do this – health professionals involved in the care of the person or friends or relatives who have engaged in activities with the person and have a sense of their capabilities.

Simplify or adapt activities. Often appropriate, this is not patronizing or infantilizing but rather a case of doing what works. It will only be patronizing or infantilizing if your manner in delivering the activity makes it so.

Look for activities that require as little mental processing as possible. You should be doing this, in general, as time goes by. Trial and error will be the order of the day, but don't rule out quite childlike intuitive activities such as throwing bean bags or patting a balloon around. Most people have a playful childish streak to their natures; people with dementia are no different.

Indeed in my view some commentators are overly sensitive when it comes to making comparisons between aspects of looking after people with dementia and young children. There are some striking similarities as well as some major differences.

It is a good idea to try to help a person with dementia keep in touch with old friends and colleagues with whom they have a shared history. In this way you will provide opportunities for activities and communication.

It is all about the here and now – your aim is to bring about a successful form of communion between the person with dementia and one or more other people at a particular time on a particular day. Don't look beyond this. Don't say a few days later, 'Did you like that game of cards we had last week?' A question like this involves a lot of mental processing. If you want to get into this for some reason, simply start talking about the activity in question, preferably with some of the artefacts involved nearby, which will then serve as a reminder.

One of the potential benefits of activities is that accompanying conversation might flow more easily and naturally than in a set piece conversation where there is a strong focus on face-to-face talking and all the pressures that can generate. The activity itself might well be the trigger for things to say.

So far as possible make sure the person uses their remaining capacities to the full. In the later stages in particular, it will often be easier to do things for people. However, this risks reminding them of how much they have lost.

One of the challenges you will encounter follows from the fact that people do not wake up one morning suddenly unable to do a particular activity. You will start to notice that a person struggles to do something they could do easily in the past. They might well become frustrated and angry with themselves. Your challenge is to judge when you need to take over the management of such activities or adapt or simplify them or stop doing them altogether.

I know a man who took great pride in writing and sending a lot of Christmas cards every year. He enclosed a number of cheques in some of them, presents for family members. A few years ago he was diagnosed with Alzheimer's disease. One year he became very confused and sent cheques to the wrong people and forgot to enclose some of the cards. The whole process made him upset and angry with himself for being 'such a useless idiot'. The family decided to turn the writing and sending of Christmas cards into a joint activity. A family member now does the organizing whilst at the same time ensuring that their relative will be as much involved as possible.

Whatever activity you do, be well prepared. Make sure you use good quality materials and if you are going to do some painting for instance make sure – in advance – that you have all the materials that you will need easily to hand. There is nothing worse than getting a person set up to do something and then spending ages messing about looking for things.

There will be times when a person does not want to engage in any activity at all. There could be a variety of reasons for this, from the drugs they are taking to general fatigue. On the basis that activities can be beneficial, persist for a while; perhaps the person will respond to a little gentle prodding. But if it is clear that they do not wish to do anything, you have to respect that without question or expressions of disappointment or regret.

If a person does not want to engage in an activity this does not necessarily mean that they do not want company.

Always remember there are times when it is pleasing and comforting to do nothing with someone, to give them a piece of your time – the simplest activity of all.

IDEAS FOR APPROPRIATE ACTIVITIES

There are countless activities which a person with dementia can do – however, it is up to you to match activities to the particular person you are caring for. Here are a few suggestions that might spark off ideas in your mind.

◆ Games
◆ Crosswords
◆ Chess
◆ Cards
◆ Painting
◆ Modelling
◆ Electric trains
◆ Knitting
◆ Cooking

The list of possibilities is endless. Ideally you will encourage and facilitate the continuation of games or hobbies the person enjoyed in the past. It might well be necessary to make adjustments – the concise crossword rather than cryptic one, draughts instead of chess, rummy or snap instead of bridge. If it becomes clear that a particular game has become too difficult and causes frustration, then simply discontinue it discreetly. Games which involve reasoning and weighing up possible options should generally be avoided.

Once a person is significantly beyond the early stages of the condition, game-type or artistic activities will probably be best on an individual (e.g. patience or a computer game aimed a people with reduced mental facilities) or one-to-one basis (a card game between the person with dementia and carer, for instance). Your assistance will be required to make things go well either as a participant or facilitator (or both).

One creative activity that seems to be particularly successful is making collages. You start with a blank bit of paper and some glue; you can then stick on pretty much anything made of paper, cardboard or light plastic – shapes, photographs from old magazines, pictures from old cereal packets, and so on. When finished, you can put them on the wall as a talking point.

In the case of drawing and painting, particularly in the later stages, a person might express feelings or concerns that it would be difficult for them to do in words – have a good look at pictures to see if they contain some underlying message.

A point worth stressing is that a person with dementia should not be mentally tested with word games or quizzes unless it is clear that they want to be; and this will only be appropriate in the early stages.

In general, putting a person with dementia under pressure in this way will cause anxiety. If you and the person do feel that such testing is appropriate and might be stimulating in a positive way, it should be limited to fairly straightforward exercises, for example:

◆ What is the capital of France?
◆ Complete this phrase, 'To err is human, to forgive . . . ?'
◆ What is the opposite of heavy?

It really all depends on the person. For some people, perhaps those with a more academic background, exercises of this kind might feel like an appropriate way of continuing to provide mental stimulation.

There are companies that produce activities from painting to jigsaws and much else besides which have been adapted for people with dementia. An online search with key words such as 'dementia activities' will take you to them. The website of the Alzheimer's Society contains much useful information.

A speech and language therapist will also be able to suggest ideas for exercises.

SUPPORT GROUPS

There might be reminiscence or other similar support groups in your area that the person with dementia could attend and which might provide conversational opportunities. In the early stages, talking to others at the same level could be particularly reassuring. Your local medical centre, speech and language therapist, occupational therapist or library should be able to give you information on what is available in your area.

Bear in mind there are support groups for carers, too – if you are helping to look after a person with dementia you might well benefit from sharing your experiences with other people.

8

Activities: Specific Examples

There are countless activities that can provide interest, stimulation and a sense of achievement for people with dementia. Nonetheless, you might feel daunted at the prospect of thinking of appropriate things to do – but the good news is that in most cases it is really just a case of adapting activities people already do or have done in the past.

MODERN TECHNOLOGY
The spectacular advances in modern technology in the last twenty or thirty years have brought benefits to people throughout the world, not least in the field of communication. Even just a comparatively short time ago, though, older people with dementia would probably not have been able to share in this bonanza. It was coming along when they already had dementia symptoms and so they would have struggled to learn the range of functions that so many people now take for granted, such as using a computer mouse or a mobile phone.

Nowadays, however, a great many people who have developed dementia in recent years were already familiar with television, video, laptops and much else when the condition started – and this will increasingly be the case in the future. With your help they can be enabled to continue using equipment of the kind they were previously familiar with.

With a little bit of imagination, you will find that much of that equipment can be transformed into valuable communicative resources. However, once more you will need to look at things from the person's point of view and make the use of modern kit as doable as possible for them.

Television

Television can be a good source of entertainment but it is not enough to turn it on and leave the person to watch it. It is better to select particular programmes that you know they will like and not be too challenged by.

◆ For so long as a person remains able to turn the television on and off independently, make sure that there is only one handset, preferably one with large, simple and intuitive keys, which is always left in the same place. Whenever you are in the room check it is in its place; if not, find it and put it there. The same goes for a CD player – and the handsets should be clearly identified 'TV' or 'CD' with a taped-on piece of paper.

◆ In general, familiar programmes will work best. *Dad's Army* is probably a good example. The person will know the characters and be amused by their antics even if, as the condition becomes more advanced, they do not follow every twist and turn of the story.

◆ Avoid dramas that involve keeping up with who did what and when, all of which involves a considerable degree of mental processing.

◆ Be wary of unpleasant subjects such as war films, gangster films or the news. A person with dementia might be disturbed by them.

◆ Programmes aimed at younger people featuring loud pop music, lots of fast banter and in-jokes are very unlikely to be pleasing to a person with dementia.

◆ As a person becomes more deeply affected by the condition they might appreciate cartoons and other children's programmes. When in the advanced stages of dementia, the sophisticated novelist Iris Murdoch derived pleasure from watching *Teletubbies*.

◆ Remember the condition is progressive and so what might have given pleasure last year might not do so this year. A person might find something to enjoy in cookery programmes even though they never did in the past. You have to keep monitoring the situation.

◆ Although not necessarily a bad thing, be aware that in the later stages a person might think that someone they see regularly on television, a friendly presenter for instance, actually comes into the house to visit them. Be sensitive. Don't correct the person but don't go along with them completely either.

Videos and DVDs

These have great possibilities, not least because you have total control over what gets shown when. This means you can set aside a time in the day or evening that best suits the person. Apart from simply watching well-loved films consider the following:

Home movies. These can be a great source of pleasing entertainment. If appropriate, you should transfer them to whatever medium makes them most user-friendly, e.g. VHS to DVD, and then show them in manageable chunks, perhaps half an hour at a time. If they are very long it might be an idea to edit them into shorter sections. Watch out for any material that might be upsetting – for instance, a deceased husband or wife or well-loved pet. You will have to monitor a person's reactions.

Record a relaxing programme. Try something on nature or oceans for instance, or a much-loved sporting event, and then play it at a time which most suits the person. As the condition progresses, you will be able to play such programmes regularly, much like playing a favourite piece of music. You might want to consider muting the sound and accompanying the film with agreeable music instead – less to process. On the other hand, it might be better to have the sound on; the lack of it might deprive the person of important information that could help them to make sense of what they are seeing on the screen.

Make your own DVDs. Perhaps the person would like to see some film of the town they grew up in or a favourite beach or hill walk that they would now be unable to undertake. You could play some well-loved music at the same time you play the film.

Arrange for close family members to be filmed talking about their memories. This could be about childhood, holidays, schooling, whatever. A person might well derive pleasure from watching this particular reminiscence group.

Put together DVDs of a person's life. Feature a lot of photographs, perhaps interspersed with some home movies and with favourite pieces of music playing in the background. You might be able to do this yourself if you are used to the technology involved. There are also companies which can perform this service.

There are organizations in America which provide DVDs aimed at people in the advanced stages of dementia. They feature a presenter who talks to the person, encourages them to do some simple exercises and talks about matters of general interest. The term used to describe these films is 'video respite'. This will not be for everybody, but there is some evidence that certain people with dementia can build up a kind of virtual relationship with the person on the screen and spend quite a long time happily watching and interacting with their screen buddy. The idea, too, is that carers have time to prepare meals or simply have a rest.

Also available are relaxing DVDs which last around fifteen or thirty minutes. For example, there is one that features a man planting some small shrubs on a beautiful sunny day. There is no narrative. Instead, the sounds of his work are clearly audible and at the same time some gentle music is playing. One person who produces such DVDs is Judi Parkinson under the title of Share-Time Pictures.

Organizations such as Memory Bank or the Scottish Screen Archive produce historical DVDs of general interest. Some of the DVDs are themed – holidays, work, home life and so on.

Do not be in any doubt that by simply facilitating and sharing any of these viewing experiences you are providing a communicative experience of quality. It might also be a good way for a visitor to spend some of their time with the person, avoiding as it does some of the pressures of face-to-face conversation.

YouTube

This brilliant phenomenon deserves a special mention. It is simple, free and opens up a window to whatever area of the past you want to take a person to.

I recently spent a wonderful hour or so with an elderly lady with dementia. We sat side by side with a laptop in front of us. I started putting in a few key names: Frank Sinatra, Gene Kelly, *The Sound of Music*, Rita Hayworth and Fred Astaire. The images burst onto the screen. The lady was transported back to happy times in the most immediate way. There were a few comments which gave an insight into her condition – 'Sinatra seems to have aged well', 'I wonder how old Fred Astaire is now', which were met with vague comments from me – it would be completely wrong to tell her that the artists in question had been dead for years.

She sang a lot of the words, moved her body in time to the music and clapped her hands. Her pleasure was unbridled.

Using a computer or tablet

Even if the person was familiar with using a computer or tablet in the past, they will almost certainly need help to initiate their use after developing dementia. In addition, since they (or you) might forget particular steps required to operate their particular bits of equipment, instructions should be printed in simple language and large font.

A quick search on the internet will take you to a great deal of interesting footage from the past – old advertisements, films of cities many years ago, clips from old television programmes, information about old warships, army regiments and much more. It is a wonderful world full of rich materials, which hold great potential for sparking off memories and conversation. You will also find remarkable things like virtual flights across America, tours of famous buildings – but do watch out in case such films cause confusion or alarm. You should do some prior research so you know in advance the suitability of what you are going to be looking at.

There are many games, such as patience or chequers, available via the internet which can be played on laptops, iPads or tablets, some of which have been specially adapted for people with impaired mental-processing powers. Touch-screen technology makes the games more user-friendly.

You could also consider setting up a private Facebook group for people who see the person with dementia on a reasonably regular basis. In this way you can keep them abreast of developments in the person's life, post photographs old and new, and make suggestions for activities that might be suitable during visits.

MUSIC

Music is relevant to many aspects of life and is discussed in Chapter 6. It can also be important as an activity. Listening to a pleasing piece of music lifts the spirits; performing music can give pleasure and allow a person to communicate emotions.

If a person played a musical instrument or participated in any singing group, then you should help them to continue with these activities for as long as possible. In addition to other benefits, it will help to boost their confidence. There will, however, probably come a point when their ability to participate will diminish; if and when it is clear that they are becoming frustrated or demoralized then the activity should be discontinued.

It is striking to notice that a person who might find it very difficult to maintain even a simple conversation can nonetheless play or sing music thoroughly learned years before. If the person has been a member of a music group, you should have a discreet word with one of the organizers. Explain the situation in the hope that you will get a sympathetic response and that allowances will be made for the person's disability.

That said, choirs and other groups do depend on a certain level of competent engagement from their members and there will come a point when a realistic decision will have to be taken. Perhaps at this stage a sympathetic friend could be asked to come and play some music at home.

A number of choirs have been set up in recent years which are specifically for people with dementia. The Alzheimer's Society helps to run a number of singing groups, featuring well-known songs from the past, under the heading 'Singing for the Brain', which have received a lot of praise from participants and their carers. If this sort of thing is of interest to you, the society will be able to advise on groups nearest to you. An internet search will help you to find choirs or music groups in your area. There are also charities, such as Nordoff Robbins, which run music workshops.

Even a person who is not particularly musical might enjoy singing some old songs, including early ones from childhood. If you are at all musical yourself it will help to make such an activity easier. Even if you are not particularly keen on singing, remember that the person will not be too bothered about the quality of your voice, and if you can overcome feelings of shyness it could be to their advantage.

A few years ago I got to know a French speech and language therapist when I lived in Nice. She let me sit in on some of the groups she ran. It never failed to amaze me how people with advanced dementia and a very limited ability to converse could nonetheless remember the words and melodies of songs they had learned many years before. They sang with real gusto and pleasure.

One specific benefit of singing is that it involves a person breathing more deeply and this leads to increased oxygenation of the blood, which can help to raise energy levels. Singing can also be associated with improved posture which, in conjunction with deeper breathing, can contribute to stronger and clearer vocal production and raised levels of alertness – all good for communication.

Music is also associated with dancing and if a person is sufficiently fit, this is an activity to encourage for the pleasure and expressiveness it produces and the contribution it can make to general physical well-being.

A great deal of recent research has stressed the benefits of physical activity for the brain.

There are some music professionals who now advocate singing as a means of helping a person to remember things they have to do each day. This will clearly not be right for everybody and it will depend on the stage a person has reached. However, imagine a person who lives alone and keeps on forgetting about daily routines. With your help a simple set of words set to a well-known tune could become an *aide-mémoire*.

> Get up in the morning, brush my teeth
> Through to the kitchen, toast and jam
> Walk to the shops, milk and bread
> Back home for lunch, cheese and ham

This might all seem banal and contrived, but if it works for the person in your life it is a potentially effective technique which can be updated from time to time.

As the condition progresses, it will be increasingly less likely that a person will be able to express themselves musically either with an instrument or their voice. At this point, listening to music will become increasingly important. You might want to consider getting a personal listening device to enable them to enjoy particular pieces of music. But these will not be suitable for everybody; some people might find the headphones and the controls a bit fiddly and uncomfortable. Your assistance will probably be required.

There is research that supports the proposition that appreciation of music continues right up to the very last stages of life. You should work on the assumption that this is true – unless you detect clear evidence of a negative response. Even if you detect little or no response, it seems highly likely that the person will derive some benefit from hearing well-loved music, including some from the very early stages of their life. Perhaps at some level it will take them back to times when they were sung to by their parents. Music can touch the inner life of a person and go straight to the emotional bloodstream in ways that are not well understood.

READING AND WRITING

It is inevitable that reading a book will become increasingly difficult for a person with dementia – very sad if this was a favourite pastime. But there are ways that with a bit of imagination reading can be maintained for a while. You should aim to find books on subjects of interest to the person, which contain a lot of pictures with simple explanations of their contents. After a while it might be that the person just looks at the pictures – which is fine: you can still talk about them.

However, the joy of reading can probably be maintained a bit longer if it becomes the joy of being read to. It is likely that you will have greatest success with books the person has read before or at least ones with subjects that are already familiar. Books with lots of characters and complex plot lines will not work. Any reading activity should be kept to reasonably short periods of time with occasional breaks.

Another possibility is poetry, or perhaps lines from songs that the person liked – and these will be freely available on the internet. The advantage here is that there are far fewer words and the message comes across quickly. There is so much available but, to give one example, the work of Pam Ayres might well be suitable.

The strong rhythms, pleasing rhymes and repetitive patterns of poetry produce a basic, almost primitive kind of creative expression, and might well be more accessible to a person with dementia than convoluted storylines. In addition, poems which a person knew earlier in life might well help to spark off memories from those times.

Contact with children and teenagers can be very pleasing for people with dementia but children can sometimes find such encounters awkward because they don't really know what to do or say. One way to counteract such difficulties would be to encourage children to bring in recent school projects – which often have lots of pictures – and tell the person about them. You should be on hand to help with clarifications or explanations.

Writing is of course an important form of communication. It becomes harder physically and mentally for most people as they get older and particularly so for people with dementia. Since there is no specific need for many people to continue writing, it is a skill that often just peters out.

You should certainly not encourage a person to write just because you think it will be a worthwhile form of brain exercise – unless you are sure they really want to.

But for some people with dementia, writing might hold rich possibilities for communication for the following reasons:

◆ It enables a person to express their feelings, concerns and observations – to give them a voice. An informal diary format might be particularly suitable. For some people of religious faith, writing simple prayers might be valuable. In addition to writing ones they are familiar with, they might write something that doesn't appear to make a great deal of sense but which might nonetheless give some insight into their thoughts.

◆ Unlike with conversation, there is no pressure to keep up with other people. It is possible to start, stop or pause at any time.

◆ Without the pressures associated with face-to-face conversation it can be easier to find the right words and phrases that reflect what the person is trying to get across.

◆ Writing can be a way of preserving a person's identity. It can also engender feelings of competence and achievement.

◆ It can also help a person to assess their current level of mental ability – although this might have the disadvantage of reminding them of their failing powers.

Writing will not be appropriate for everybody. It might be most suitable for people who have been used to writing in the past, perhaps as part of their work. Your assistance will be required to provide materials, give feedback and give encouragement for an activity which could also provide valuable opportunities for conversation.

One alternative to physically writing things down would be for you to record what the person says on a dictating machine or by using your smartphone and then transcribe it at a later date.

CARING FOR PETS

A person with dementia will find it increasingly difficult to look after a pet if they live on their own. This can be a significant loss for people who have shared much of their lives with an animal. As many people know, animals are capable of generating feelings of pleasure, companionship and satisfaction that can be profound and which require no mental processing at all. They also allow a person to express things about themselves.

I did some voluntary work in a care home near Cannes a few years ago. There was one elderly woman who regularly sat out on the terrace. She had dementia. She never smiled and always looked worried and fretful. One day her daughter arrived with her small dog. The transformation in the woman was unbelievable. She became animated, smiled and made many sounds of pleasure as she patted the dog. There were hardly any actual words spoken. I thought what a shame it would have been if she had not had this opportunity to communicate such attractive aspects of her personality. I'm sure a lot of people casually thought of her as grumpy and uninterested in life, fading away in the sun.

In the early stages, with a little bit of support from you, it might be possible for a person to continue to have a pet at home, but this will not be feasible in the long term. You could consider the possibility of visits to or from people with cats or dogs. Perhaps the person could accompany a neighbour when taking their dog out for a walk.

In these ways a person could still experience at least some of the positive messages that animals can communicate without the responsibility of looking after them.

Alzheimer Scotland has recently been involved in the setting up of a scheme to provide 'dementia dogs'. The dogs are trained to help people with dementia – not just by providing companionship but also other things such as reminding them to take medicine. There will doubtless be more initiatives like this in the future.

Consider also a tropical fish tank which can be an excellent source of interest and stimulation – and there are no daily walks.

HOUSEHOLD ACTIVITIES

It is likely that a person with dementia ran or helped to run a household for many years, taking responsibilities for many aspects of day-to-day life. As dementia progresses a person will gradually lose the desire and the ability to keep on doing this. However, it is important that the person is not given the message that everything should suddenly come to a juddering halt. Some carers might seek to dress this up as a good thing – no more work, a chance to sit and relax with the paper. But while some people might welcome this many won't as it could engender feelings of uselessness and disempowerment.

Also, just because they cannot do everything does not mean they cannot do something.

Try to find ways to enable them to continue doing at least part of the work. If you are cooking a meal set things up for the person to peel vegetables or lay the table, and overlook or discreetly correct any mistakes. If you are doing some washing the person could help with folding and putting away. It all depends on the stage of the person's dementia and, as always, you will have to monitor and facilitate – frustrating when you know you could do everything much more quickly on your own.

If the person in question is one of your parents, what happens is a gradual role reversal from the time when you were young.

Try to see daily activities as communication opportunities. Make some meals you know the person cooked in the past. Talk about the ingredients – you might find out how much they cost back in the day. When making meals, ask the person to taste the food as it is cooking and get their reaction – much of this can be done with gestures and hand signals. It is all about maintaining and respecting the abilities the person retains.

You might also find that though a person will not understand how to work a modern washing machine they will nonetheless remember clearly how clothes were washed in the past – could you recreate this and talk about it? This kind of thinking applied to any number of household, or indeed gardening, jobs might prove fruitful.

SOCIAL OCCASIONS

Get-togethers with friends and relatives can be a double-edged experience for a person with dementia. Like most people they get a lot of pleasure from such meetings. However, a person with dementia will invariably find it hard to follow a conversation involving several people. The chances are the noise of lots of people talking will quickly become meaningless and likely to cause feelings of exclusion. It will be hard for the person to contribute. That said, they will still want to be part of the proceedings.

A bit of forward planning can help to ensure that such occasions go well. One-to-one conversations will be far easier for a person with dementia to participate in. With a few phone calls in advance, try to ensure that visitors are aware of this. Set aside an area of a room, or a separate room, where such conversations can take place and make sure they do.

If a person will be meeting someone they have not seen for a while or have not met before, try to prepare them with some key points about the new person and why they will be seeing them – and do this a couple of times or more, once not long before the meeting takes place.

People sometimes worry about children meeting people with dementia. But a brief and simplified explanation about the person's condition together with advice about not making too much noise – which can be distracting and alarming – should be sufficient to ensure that meetings with children go smoothly.

In the case of youngsters, it is often a case of the simple pleasure of watching them do whatever children do, perhaps from a distance if the play is boisterous.

Although it might not happen very often, meeting a person from a foreign country – even someone who was well known in the past – can present its own challenges. Hearing a foreign language, or English, spoken with a strong foreign accent, particularly in the later stages, can be confusing. Assuming the person has not been abroad for quite a while it could be difficult to match up the sounds of a foreign language with the parts of their memory where this information is stored. If possible, show the person some old photographs of the visitor before the meeting and talk about the country in question and the way people speak there.

OUTINGS

The majority of activities a person with dementia engages in will probably take place indoors. Yet there is also much to be said for outdoor occasions. If you have a garden or access to a nearby park, then when the weather allows, a person with dementia will almost certainly benefit from the opportunity to watch the many seemingly everyday things that can be observed – from workmen digging up the road to children playing on the slide. Such everyday things are often taken for granted but they can provide a lot of visual stimulation and pleasure.

Activities which involve travelling longer distances – visits to friends or relatives, for instance – might also be desirable, but there can be pitfalls.

I knew a man whose mother had been diagnosed with vascular dementia some years previously. The condition was well advanced and though she was quite fit physically, she was easily confused about many aspects of day-to-day life. Her son decided that he wanted to do something special for her birthday. He took a week off work and arranged to take her to visit three relatives in different parts of England. This trip involved a lot of travelling, a lot of changes of scene, and a lot of meetings with people, some of whom his mother had not seen for several years.

The whole thing was a disaster. His mother was totally confused and unsettled by the trip and was often very agitated and tearful. She really did not understand what was going on much of the time. Her son was upset that his good intentions and planning had resulted in such an unhappy outcome. He kept on saying how much his mother had always enjoyed such trips in the past.

He had not taken on board some of the most important aspects of helping to care for and communicate with a person with dementia: the old ways won't work; change is necessary. The person cannot change – so you have to.

Though well-intentioned, the son went about things in the wrong way. Change and transitions become increasingly difficult for a person with dementia, and creating several in a short space of time was too much for his mother to cope with. I have even heard of people considering jetting off to some far-off country so that a person can see a particular relative one last time. This kind of thinking fails to put the person first and will almost certainly produce high levels of stress and agitation.

So what should the son in the above scenario have done? There is no absolutely correct answer to this question. But there are things he could have done . . .

- At the start of his week off, he could have arranged for one relative to visit his mother at her own home.

- Shortly prior to the relative's arrival he could have told his mother about the visit, shown her a few photographs, explored some of his own memories of the person in the hope that this sparked off some memories for his mother, too.

- Prior to the relative's arrival, he could have made a phone call – not in his mother's presence – to make the visitor aware of her up-to-date condition and advise on some important points, e.g. allowing plenty of time for his mother to say what she had to say and not quizzing or contradicting her.

- Thereafter, he might have considered a short trip later in the week to whichever of the other relatives lived nearest.

◆ Once more he could have shown his mother some photographs shortly before the trip and had a discreet phone call with the relative.

If you ever think of laying on some outing for a person with dementia you should look at the whole thing from their point of view. As the condition progresses, they will find upheaval and change unsettling and stressful. You might think it's a really nice idea to go to the zoo or the fairground or to visit Auntie Jane at the other end of the country, but just visualize all the steps that the person with dementia has to go through from start to finish and all the things they will experience along the way. The chances are that each one will involve something that is not part of the person's normal everyday routine and which might be upsetting for them.

I am not saying you should never take people out on trips – far from it; they can be pleasant and stimulating. However, I am saying that you should keep them – so far as possible – simple, short and familiar, particularly when the condition becomes more advanced. Perhaps there is a garden centre or a country house nearby that you could start visiting from time to time.

A trip like this – getting there, walking about, seeing some interesting things, having a bowl of soup and then getting back to base, might all take three to four hours. Ideal.

This would mean the person would still have the secure framework of all of their regular morning and evening routines. This is only one example – I don't know the person in your life, but I hope you get the picture. A good idea would be to have a small repertoire of such trips that you can do over and over again. If they are successful once, they almost certainly will be again.

Here are a few more points to consider about outings:

Consider visits to places that were of importance during a person's life – old work places, schools, former houses – but bear in mind that such visits will be most appropriate for people in the early stages. Later on, such visits could cause confusion or it might simply be the case that they will not bring back memories as you had hoped.

Plan ahead. Visit places you think might be suitable and check that any café or restaurant is reasonably dementia-friendly; that toilets are easily accessible and that there are some pleasant areas for gentle strolling. Bear in mind, too, that the noise of coffee machines and children's play areas can be very distracting for a person with dementia – choose seats as far away from these hazards as possible. Consider taking some photographs to show to the person shortly prior to the visit.

Don't feel that an outing must always involve doing lots of things. Simply going to watch, for instance, a local cricket match can be a worthwhile activity on various levels. Apart from watching something reasonably interesting but undemanding there will be opportunities to chat. Above all you are giving the person the most important thing of all – your company.

When you go on an outing take a few photographs. Print them off when you get home; a good trigger for conversation.

However, when you are looking at them later and talking about them remember: *Tell don't ask.*

Dementia cafés. The Alzheimer's Society and other dementia charities run and support specialized cafés. The idea is that people can go there with relatives or friends, meet and talk to other people and also receive information and support from trained advisers.

Think of activities that involve several senses. In the garden for instance, encourage the person to rub the leaf of a herb between their fingers and enjoy the scent. If you buy apples in a shop, make an apple pie with the person's assistance – coring, peeling and chopping the apples perhaps.

Be aware of festivals or celebrations throughout the year. Try to tie activities in with them – particularly ones which have been significant in the person's life.

Capitalize on things the person has done regularly in the past. For instance, some people will have had a daily ritual of collecting a newspaper on the way to or from work. This could be adapted so that they walk to and from the local newsagent on a regular basis – with your or somebody else's assistance if necessary.

Bear in mind that a person might enjoy the continuity of such an activity, even if their ability to make sense of the newspaper is limited to following a few headlines or looking at pictures and recognizing some familiar faces.

Similarly, going to the shops can be a very simple but pleasing activity. It is all about the person continuing to do things they have always done. Familiar and reassuring things.

Nevertheless, do apply common sense when you get back home – don't leave the person to put the shopping away. Trying to remember where everything goes might well involve too much memory consultation. Make the process a joint activity.

One particular activity to consider which is simple, cheap and potentially very stimulating is people watching. Countless tourists on foreign holidays derive a huge amount of pleasure from doing this – as well as its close relative, soaking up the atmosphere. The important thing here is to make sure the location is right. Outdoor cafés or parks where there are a lot of people moving around are ideal.

When it comes to activities the preferences of the person should generally be paramount; but if you can come up with things that you happen to like as well – visiting a new country house, for instance – all the better.

In the advanced stages of dementia a person will become less and less interested in many of the kinds of activities discussed in this chapter. You just have to accept this and try to create an environment that contains and generates sounds, sights or aromas which are capable of reaching the person directly.

This might be favourite music or even something as basic as placing the person's chair in front of a window that looks out on to a scene of interest – a road, a park or a cityscape of rooftops.

It will be hard to tell to what extent such stimuli enhance a person's life. Do things that, based on previous experience, you think will work and look for any signs, however small, of positive or negative reactions and respond accordingly.

9

Aids to Memory and Communication

When a person's eyesight or hearing starts to deteriorate, it's quite simple to deal with – you get glasses or hearing aids to keep these vital channels of communication operating as efficiently as possible for as long as possible. When the memory stops working effectively, however, it is more difficult; the brain is so much more complex. But there are many ways in which artificial aids can be brought into play to help compensate for the problems caused by a failing memory and reduced cognitive abilities.

USING PICTURES, NOTICES AND SIGNS

There are countless ways you can cut down the amount of mental processing a person with dementia needs to do in their home environment. Information in the form of written signs and pictures has the greatest potential to help during the middle stages of dementia. In the early stages they will probably not be necessary – and might risk being seen as patronizing. In the later stages the person might have difficulty making sense of anything other than very simple pictures.

When you do put up signs make sure that they do not become dog-eared – renew them every now and then. It is a good idea to laminate them. If you make any changes try to keep the signs looking similar to the way they were previously – avoid radical change.

The following list contains some suggestions and comments. However, before you do anything, there are a number of points to bear in mind:

◆ Make sure the font is the right size for the person to read easily.

◆ Keep templates on your laptop so that they can easily be updated.

◆ Keep the number of words used to an absolute minimum.

◆ Ensure there is a marked contrast between the letters and the background to make the words stand out as much as possible.

◆ Consider including pictures as well as words.

◆ Make sure that the words used are straightforward and unambiguous.

◆ Ensure that any notices are close to the thing they relate to and are at a height that can be seen easily by the person with dementia.

◆ Don't introduce such things because you think in theory it sounds like a good idea – only do it if you have reason to believe the person will benefit.

◆ Use trial and error to see what works best – everyone is different.

So what kind of things should you consider putting up on the wall?

Diaries and calendars

Diaries and calendars are great for day-to-day events and are particularly valuable in the early stages. However, a person with dementia might still need to be prompted to check them – either by you in person or on the phone. If a person lives alone visitors should be encouraged to check the diary with the person when they arrive. They need to be updated regularly in order to maintain their relevance and usefulness.

Pictures

Select pictures of people who visit regularly – family members, close friends and health professionals. Choose an area of a wall in a part of the house that is easily accessible. Alternatively, you could create a file or folder. Such pictures can help to prepare a person for a visit: rather than just telling them about a visit, reinforce the verbal message with a picture – and do it all as one action so that maximum clarity is achieved. Next to each picture should be the person's name together with brief essential information – 'Jean's daughter', 'Doctor', 'Care assistant'.

One thing to bear in mind, though – if some of the friends or family in the photographs do not visit very often, then photographs might serve to underline this fact.

Update your choices from time to time.

Activity list

You could have a list of favourite activities prominently displayed somewhere – certain ones on certain days, perhaps with some accompanying photographs, of a park or a café or whatever. These will serve as reminders and also prompts for visitors who might be looking for ideas for things to do.

Labels

A person with dementia might start to forget which items are in which drawers. Labels, perhaps with simple pictures, will help to communicate this information and thus avoid the need to try to remember. Further on it might well be helpful to put signs/pictures on the doors to particular rooms.

Signs for particular purposes

If, for example, you live with a person with dementia or are a live-in carer and need to go out for a while, confusion can occur. Despite having been given an explanation, the person with dementia might forget after a short time that you had to go out and start to panic. To prevent this happening, a simple sign on the inside of the front door or some other prominent place – 'Malcolm, gone to shops – back soon' – might be just enough to defuse the situation.

You could also consider setting up a sign that gives the current day, month, year, the person's address, town/city, the weather forecast – which would help to orient the person. This would of course require constant updating. There are electrically or battery-operated clocks available, which contain and update some of this information automatically – but they would have to have large letters and numbers.

There are new products coming onto the market all the time and it is a good idea to do internet searches from time to time and to follow up on reports you hear on news programmes.

Instructions and reminders

The need for such instructions and reminders will depend on the person and the stage of the condition they have reached. Simple diagrams with instructions for how to operate a coffee machine, CD player, laptop, washing machine, the brake on a wheelchair, immersion heater – and much else besides – could just help to avoid difficulties if a person, particularly if they live alone, forgets some basic instruction. You could also have magnetized stickers on the fridge with reminders about having drinks or preparing food regularly.

Communicating information in this way can help to avoid confusion and frustration and also allow a person to have a little bit more independence.

Similarly, dosette boxes that are loaded up with a person's pills for a period of time, and which are split up into compartments for each day of the week, can be very helpful. That said, the person cannot be expected to put the pills in the compartments and supervision will be required to ensure that the pills are being taken at appropriate times.

Information cards

When a person is still able go out alone, it is probably a good idea for them to carry an easily accessible card with a few important details – first name, a couple of contact numbers and some basic information, for instance: 'Mike has a condition which means he has problems with his memory and he needs time to answer questions.' This could perhaps be contained in some kind of bracelet that would be visible to a member of the public. With information like this readily available you might feel the person can go out alone for a bit longer.

Around the house

Smoke/carbon monoxide alarms/panic buttons/ doorbells

◆ Although there is a very real risk of fear and upset being caused when alarms go off, if a person with dementia lives alone such devices are vital. To put it bluntly, people with dementia are more likely to forget to switch off the heat under a pan. The alarms communicate to the person that there is a problem that needs addressing urgently. At the very least, there is an increased chance that the person will phone you or press a personal alarm or panic button and get help.

◆ A panic button can be problematic because a person might not want to wear it, forget to put it on or press it inappropriately. But if a person lives alone you really should consider this potentially life-saving form of communication.

◆ You should ensure that the doorbell is sufficiently loud and long-lasting for a person living on their own to be able to hear it clearly. Regular visitors will be aware that the person might need some extra time to come to the door but other visitors might not. Accordingly, it is a good idea to put a discreet sign next to the doorbell advising callers that the person needs a little extra time to come to the door.

◆ For some people a digital clock might be easier to understand than a more old-fashioned clock, although many will prefer the familiarity of the old.

Rooms

Furniture and room layout can be modified or adapted in such a way as to transmit valuable information to a person with dementia. For instance:

Knowing what is in a cupboard or a fridge or a wardrobe is a question of memory. Glass doors in these units, preferably lit up (possibly by sensors), mean that they communicate their contents with minimal mental processing on the part of a person with dementia.

If you paint doors a particular colour this will help to identify which rooms they lead to – bathroom, kitchen, bedroom; and this can of course be backed up with words or pictures. Negotiating houses with such cues will be easier for a person with dementia. The use of contrasting colours is likely to be beneficial.

Where possible, doors should be left open – so that the person can identify rooms with a brief glance.

Thinking about things in this way is all part of the knack of looking at things from the point of view of the person and coming up with ideas for making changes that work.

Ideally, a person with dementia should be able to see their bathroom from their bed. An ensuite is perfect; a light left on, with the door open during the night, will make it much easier for the person to get there in time. Of course most bedrooms do not have ensuite facilities. You could consider rigging up a rope or brightly coloured strip of paper along the wall from the bedroom door to the bathroom. You can also buy nightlights which can be plugged into wall sockets. Some people have found that having a brightly coloured toilet seat makes accidents less likely.

When a person has visitors, think about the position of their chair. In the early stages this will not be particularly important, but it can be later on. If you put a person in a central position they will symbolically be at the heart of things. They will certainly get more attention – but they will also have people talking all around them. Which one will they try to tune into? Will they be able to concentrate on what one of a number of people is saying to them?

If you place them off to the side they will be in a kind of observer role and it might be that this will be absolutely right for some people – happy to engage in some family or friends people watching but not at the centre of things and not expected to contribute too much. People can then approach the person and have one-to-one conversations. However, the noise of the other people in the room could be very distracting and so perhaps it would be better to set up a couple of chairs face-to-face in another room for such encounters.

There is really no right or wrong answer – it will depend on particular situations and particular people. Always try to put yourself in the place of the person with dementia and try to work out what would feel best for them, based on your knowledge of them and their current capabilities.

AIDS TO STIMULATE MEMORY AND CONVERSATION

Photograph albums

Looking through family photograph albums can provide many opportunities for fruitful activities based on reminiscence. However, there are a number of points to bear in mind:

◆ When looking at photographs do not turn the activity into a quiz: 'Who's that standing next to Uncle David? Surely you remember her?' *Tell don't ask.*

◆ If you think the person might have some information they want to contribute, start talking about the pictures and the people in them and see if this triggers some memories.

◆ Take care, so far as possible, not to produce photographs or any other memorabilia that might have unhappy associations and upset the person.

◆ Be prepared. Go through photographs yourself first and note down as much information as possible – the people, the places, the occasion – so that you can provide details as you go through them. Choose clear, non-blurry photographs where the people are easy to make out, and only have one or two photographs per page.

◆ If the person asks specific questions about the photographs, be fairly vague in your responses, as the people in them might be dead or unwell – 'It was quite a few years ago', 'Haven't seen John for a while'.

◆ Try to broaden the communicative possibilities. For instance if looking at old photographs draw attention to the fashions, the cars, the shops – and be specific – 'There's an old Hillman Hunter . . . you had one like that, a blue one.' In this way you might prompt the person to produce some comments of their own.

◆ The very nature of dementia means that you can bring out the same photographs from time to time – particularly ones you know have generated interest and pleasure previously.

Memory albums

The idea of this kind of album is to include souvenirs and memorabilia from the past – a menu, concert tickets, a programme, headed paper of the company where the person worked, travel documents – whatever might, with your help, spark memories and conversation.

There are products available commercially; an online search will take you to companies that have templates and blank albums of various kinds which you can then personalize. These might work well, but with a little imagination it is not hard to put together something yourself, which will be created with just one person in mind.

Whatever you do, you should occasionally update any albums you produce. Photos of a relative or well-loved pet that has died since the album was originally put together might, for example, be better removed. Also, photos taken on successful outings that have taken place could be added.

Real objects

In a similar vein, some people have what they call rummage boxes – the size of the box and the contents are entirely a matter of personal choice. The contents might include an old childhood toy, a book, a stamp album, a piece of jewellery, a school report, work tools, souvenirs from family holidays in Spain, miniature pictures – it really could be anything. Stuff that works.

People should be encouraged to hold and feel the objects. If possible try to recreate aromas or scents associated with some of the objects – smell has a powerful ability to bring back memories of places or feelings from the past.

*Interestingly, some people – who do not have dementia – are
already putting together their own rummage boxes in case they
should ever develop dementia in later life. They want to be sure
that the box contains things that are right for them.*

Dolls or comfort toys

This is an area that can be controversial. It is relevant to people
in the more advanced stages of dementia and may be more so to
those in residential care homes – though there is no particular
reason why such objects should not be used in the family home.

The idea is that a person is introduced to a doll or other soft toy
to which they become attached – holding it, talking to it, talking
about it to other people, taking it for walks in the garden, and so
on. The introduction of the doll should be handled sensitively.
It might be best to leave it lying on the person's bed or to hold it
yourself and sit next to the person with the doll clearly in view.
You might then start to interact with it yourself and hope that the
person gradually shows an interest and then takes it from you –
something you should do your best to make as natural and easy
as possible. Some people won't be interested.

It might be that the doll sparks off feelings and thoughts from
the past. Perhaps it is simply the case that people with advanced
dementia find that attachment to a doll satisfies a basic need to
protect and care for a helpless 'being'; or it could be that they just
like the look and the feel of it. What is certain is that in some
nursing homes where dolls have been introduced, there has been
a significant degree of success – measurable in terms of reduced
anxiety levels, contented behaviour and in some cases a radical
reduction in the number of drugs taken by the person. Some
relatives have spoken of people getting a new lease of life.

With advances in technology, robotic pets have been developed. A Japanese scientist has developed an attractive-looking baby seal (not specifically aimed at people with dementia) with multiple sensors under its fur – which responds to touch and stroking much as a cat or a dog would. For some people with dementia these devices are already providing comfort and pleasure and it is likely that more and more products of this kind will come on to the market, although at the present time they are still very expensive.

Some people see dolls or robotic pets for adults as inappropriate on the basis that it is a case of treating them like children. While there are parallels with the way young children relate to favourite dolls or comfort toys, it is surely a question of judging the idea by its results.

If it is clear that a person derives genuine comfort and pleasure from having a doll or robotic pet, who is to say this is wrong simply on the basis of some intellectual or theoretical fear of treating the person like a child?

That said, it might be hard to watch a much-loved relative, who ran a business or held down a responsible job, behave in this way. This though is all part of the kind of radical change of outlook you need to make in order to do the best for a person with dementia.

Talking Mats

This is a straightforward low-tech aid to communication that involves a person expressing views on various topics by placing symbols in appropriate places on a mat. It is appropriate for people in the later stages of dementia when conversation and reasoning has become significantly impaired. An aid generally administered by professionals who have had some training, there is, however, no reason why the basic techniques could not be utilized by anybody.

Although it is not specifically aimed at enabling conversation, the very process of carrying it out will involve focused interaction between the person with dementia and whoever is facilitating – a potentially enjoyable and stimulating experience for the person.

Talking Mats could well be helpful in a situation where the opinion of a person with fairly advanced dementia is sought. This might be in connection with their care or perhaps a legal issue, or indeed to help assess their current level of mental capacity. It might be there are concerns that a person is suffering in some way but is unable to express this clearly. One research project found that the system was more effective in allowing a person to express views about their well-being, and things happening in their lives, than a more conventional question and answer session. The nature of Talking Mats means that there is plenty of time for a person to formulate views without the normal pressures of spoken conversation.

Talking Mats involves the use of a textured mat which measures around eighteen inches by twelve. At the top are three permanent symbols representing respectively:

Good/I like it
Neutral/I'm not really sure
Bad/I don't like it

A selection of pictures/symbolic representations of aspects of a person's life are then produced. These are placed under the symbol at the top of the mat that accords with the person's view. For instance, if the person places a photograph of food under the *Bad/I don't* like it symbol, then you know the food offered to the person needs to be reconsidered.

The system would have to be demonstrated and explained to the person and you would need to be satisfied that they understood what was expected of them. If you created a mat covering a number of topics, you could photograph it and use it as a reference point in the future to see how particular things have changed over time. Such pictures might also be helpful for health professionals involved in the care of the person.

If the Talking Mats technique is introduced earlier rather than later, it might mean that later on, once a person's condition has progressed, the technique could provide a valuable way for them to express views in a way that is already familiar.

Note, too, that a digital version of Talking Mats is available.

Talking Mats will probably only be appropriate for a small minority of people with dementia. However, it is another tool in the armoury for helping to improve communication in some situations and might be worthy of your consideration. A speech and language therapist involved in the care of a person with dementia will be able to give further guidance.

One simple variation could be to produce some photographs or flash cards of areas of a person's life and then use non-verbal gestures such as thumbs-up or thumbs-down to elicit the person's feelings.

Talking Mats is just one example of an aid to communication which has been devised by professionals to make communication with people with impaired mental powers easier. A speech and language therapist will be able to advise you about others.

10

Dealing with Difficult Situations

All serious health conditions produce their own set of difficulties and challenges. Dementia is no exception. It interferes with and impairs the workings of the brain and this can lead to behaviour and actions that can cause frustration, and indeed despair, on the part of people who help to look after them, particularly as the condition progresses towards the later stages.

There are many strategies which can make communication easier and help to reduce stress. Sometimes, however, the challenges you are faced with can seem particularly hard to overcome.

There is one thing you should keep telling yourself: it is the condition that makes them do what they do. If you can keep on reminding yourself of this it might help to keep you on an even keel when the going gets tough.

I have occasionally heard people say that a relative with dementia was putting it on, deliberately trying to make their lives difficult, pretending not to understand things said to them when really they did. Even if there is a little bit of truth in such assertions, the reality is that the principal cause of any difficult behaviour is the condition. Perhaps the person does have faults – doesn't everyone? – but they are in trouble and they need your help.

The fact is that once the professionals have carried out a series of assessments – a process which might last two years or so – and concluded that a person has, or probably has, dementia, you have to accept this and adjust to the new future that confronts you.

Here are some examples of frequently encountered situations.

ASKING THE SAME QUESTIONS REPEATEDLY

In all stages, but particularly in the more advanced stage, the person will probably not remember that they have already asked the question. They might also forget that their son's wife never drinks coffee and offer it every time she visits. Despite inevitable and understandable feelings of exasperation there is no point in telling the person that they have already asked the same question thirty times since breakfast; nor correcting them about somebody's dislike of coffee. Nothing will be achieved beyond raising stress levels.

Sometimes there will be an underlying message. You might be able to uncover this by taking some time, sitting with the person, and trying to play back some of the key phrases they use in order to get beyond the small group of words used in the repetitive questions.

For example, if a person continually asks whether gas bills have been paid, it might be that they are feeling cold. It might also be an expression of anxiety over a loss of control over their financial affairs. In either case, engaging with the person in a calm atmosphere free from distractions might reveal the underlying concern. It might then be a case of getting another pullover or reassuring the person about finances.

If a person forgets that they have recently had a meal and continually asks about having some food, you could tell them that they had eaten recently and that the next meal will not be for a couple of hours. This would, however, achieve little and the questions would doubtless start again soon. A better strategy would be to have a few light snacky things available, give a vague assurance that a meal will soon be on the way and then try to divert the person with an activity or a change of scene.

If a person in a care home continually asks when their daughter will be visiting, it might simply mean they feel lonely and would like some company – taking a little time to sit and chat might help to ease things.

For people who ask the same questions regularly you could consider having some sheets of paper with certain key bits of information providing the answers in a few words. Then, in response to the questions, you could point the person in the direction of the sheets, which could be contained in a folder or receptacle in a prominent place in the living room, and hope that they will subsequently be able to refer to them without prompting. This involves a level of processing and would probably not work when the condition is more advanced. It would probably be a good idea to go through the sheets with the person from time to time, even when they are not asking the questions.

Sometimes there is no strategy that will work and it is probably best just to smile, be patient, give the appropriate answer calmly and try to engage in any activity that will help to divert the person's focus elsewhere.

LOOKING FOR THINGS

If a person with dementia can't find something, they can become determined and single-minded in their search for it. It can be hard or impossible to deflect them from their quest, let alone engage in conversation or other activity. Such episodes might reflect a powerful feeling of loss of control or competence or a sense of losing grip on their ability to be in charge of their lives. Responses such as, 'It doesn't matter, I'm sure it will turn up' might offer momentary comfort but no more. Then again, you do not want to find yourself regularly spending the whole afternoon hunting high and low for a key.

Initially it is probably best to engage in a calmly conducted search in likely places, all the while allowing the person to express their frustrations at their inability to find the missing object.

However, as you do this, think of ways the person can be diverted – a cup of tea, a trip to the shops, going through to a room where there are some objects of interest, so that the process of searching – assuming the item is not found – can be brought to an end with the person moving away from their frustrating thoughts within a reasonable length of time.

Check now and then that items that are of particular importance – glasses, keys, a handbag, hearing aids – are in the right place. Prevention is better than cure.

DRIVING

The ability to drive a car is an expression of independence that many of us take for granted. We all know there will come a point when we will have to give it up and will gradually adjust to that. But in the case of people with dementia, the moment to give up comes sooner and it might well be that the person does not really understand or indeed accept the need to lose such a large amount of freedom. The impact can be particularly acute for couples where the person who loses the ability to drive is the sole driver.

As and when you become aware that a person has or probably has dementia, you need to consider the question of how long they can continue driving. You should keep a close eye on any incidents or near misses, which might indicate that driving is becoming dangerous.

In the early stages it might be perfectly safe for them to drive for a while. That said, you should gradually ensure that the amount and the kind of drives they take is adjusted appropriately – no long journeys on motorways, no night driving; move towards just driving well-known routes to the local shops or nearby friends.

However, you have to weigh up the possible danger to the person and, of course, other road users. A person with dementia is unlikely to volunteer to stop driving. Family members, after consultation with medical advisers, are usually the ones who take the final decision – which might be the result of some near misses, a bump, a scrape or just a strong feeling that the situation cannot continue.

In approaching the issue you really do need to show sensitivity. It is quite likely you will be telling your parent that an activity they have been doing for years is now no longer available to them.

This represents quite a shift – in the distant past, and for many years, the relationship was the other way around. It is likely the person will feel some resentment.

◆ Avoid being critical of the person.

◆ Diplomatically draw attention to any incidents or near misses with a view to persuading the person it is the right decision.

◆ You want to avoid damaging your relationship with the person and so you should shift responsibility on to the person's medical advisers or the DVLA.

Try to avoid giving the impression that it is you who is making the person give up driving.

Once a person has a diagnosis of dementia, the DVLA (DVLNI in Northern Ireland) has to be informed. This does not mean that the person is automatically barred from driving but it does mean that a form will have to be completed giving details of their current situation; they might have to undergo a practical test to assess their current level of ability and whether they can continue to drive.

Think of alternatives to driving – such as lifts from family or friends, bus trips, rail journeys or taxis – and promote the merits of these alternatives.

Once you are certain that the person cannot safely continue to drive you will need to take some practical steps such as hiding the keys, disabling the car or indeed selling it.

Some people believe that even at this stage the person should be allowed to keep their old driving licence in a wallet as a kind of symbol of independence.

TELLING THE TRUTH

There is some controversy surrounding the question of whether or not it is acceptable to lie to a person with dementia. We live in a world where, in theory at least, transparency and openness have become elevated to gold-standard benchmarks in many areas of life. However, to apply such standards rigidly to all day-to-day dealings with a person with dementia would be both unrealistic and counter-productive. Earlier examples have demonstrated how it is possible to come up with strategies that do not duck issues but which stop short of telling the whole truth. Even if this is morally questionable, I believe this is a great deal more morally acceptable than inflicting avoidable emotional suffering on the person.

It should not be forgotten that when a person with dementia thinks, for instance, that a dead relative is currently at work, they are not making it up; they believe it at the time they say it. There might be other times when they do understand the true situation – dementia does not happen evenly and logically. If you try to pull the person out of their reality by correcting them, you risk causing some upset and will almost certainly not achieve anything positive.

You might seek to defend yourself by claiming that you were simply telling the truth, but that is a cop-out, one that avoids coming up with a more constructive approach.

Having said all that, it is very doubtful whether wholeheartedly agreeing with or going along with a mistaken belief on the part of the person is generally a good idea. If a person wants to know when their mother, who died ten years previously, will be coming home, you could say, 'She's at the shops, she'll be back in half an hour', in the hope that the person will forget about it.

Such responses might provide temporary relief, but there are questions to be asked:

> *Would you then have to get other relatives, friends or carers to go along with the ploy? If so you would have to make sure you were all saying the same thing. What if they did not agree with engaging in this kind of deception?*

> *Is it acceptable to use the person's impaired memory to manipulate difficult situations?*

> *Although the person's memory is badly impaired perhaps they will realize that they are being duped, which might undermine whatever trust they have in you or other carers?*

As a general rule it is best to try to enter into what is real for the person at a particular time, to empathize, prompt the person to express memories and feelings – without actually confirming that a mistaken statement is true – and then look for an opportunity to divert them towards another activity. You should certainly not simply ignore untrue statements by the person, but it is doubtful that there is anything to be gained from shattering illusions which might well pass in a short time.

The situation is not black and white and you should reflect on the subject and discuss it with other people in the hope you will develop a knack for responding effectively as and when situations arise.

I am in no doubt there are times when it is acceptable to be economical with the truth or to exercise a little deception for the greater good. Some people use the expression 'therapeutic lies'.

Here are a few more instances:

- If a person is particularly agitated about something they think they need to do – deliver an item to a customer, for example – you could say that somebody else has already done it and they can do it next time. This is a white lie about something that is much less important than information about, for instance, whether a close relative is alive or dead.

- If you think a person with dementia who lives alone is not eating enough, you could arrive with some soup or stew. You could say that you had made too much and that it would be a pity to waste it. You could make it appear that the person was doing you a favour. A minor deception in a good cause.

- If a person is attached to a particular item of clothing which they associate with going out but you know that the item in question – shoes with holes, a lightweight coat – will be inappropriate or inadequate, then prevention will almost certainly be the best course. Make sure the items in question are put safely away somewhere and then produce more-appropriate items; in this way you will hope to avoid the person putting on the wrong things, which you then have to get them to change.

One particularly difficult situation is whether to tell a person with dementia about the death of a close friend or relative. This raises tricky questions such as:

Do they not have a right to know?
Should they be protected from emotional pain in all
   circumstances?

The guiding principle here will probably be the stage their condition has reached. In the very late stages there is almost certainly nothing to be gained. However, in the earlier stages the principle that the person has a right to know is surely paramount. The difficult part is deciding about the bits in between. They might well realize that you are upset about something and so keeping the information from them might create difficulties.

This will be a matter of judgement for you based on your knowledge of the person; you should also consider talking to other close family and friends as well as health professionals.

If a person is upset and agitated about, for instance, friends and relatives not coming to visit, don't be dismissive and say something which, though vague, is not definitely true: 'Oh it's OK, I think your grandson is coming next week some time.' This will probably not provide much comfort. It would be far better to sit down and encourage them to talk about the person in question and, for instance, places they have visited together – these are the kinds of things that will be in the person's mind and you will be helping them to express pleasant memories and feelings.

DISTURBED AND AGGRESSIVE BEHAVIOUR

There are times, particularly in the more advanced stages, when a person with dementia can suddenly become very upset or agitated for reasons that are not immediately obvious. This can lead to disruptive behaviour. The person might shout, scream, hit out or bite. They are certainly communicating something but the nature of the message can be very hard to glean.

The person might:

◆ Be angry about their personal space being invaded during care procedures.

◆ Feel extreme frustration at their lack of ability to communicate.

◆ Feel ashamed or inadequate.

◆ Be experiencing a hallucination.

◆ Be experiencing pain.

The person's condition can make it very hard for them to express their feelings in conventional ways. Urgent situations – often associated with bathing, getting undressed or other intimate procedures – can arise out of the blue.

With regard to bathing and showering, bear in mind that many older people were brought up at a time when people had baths less frequently than they do now. Also, showers were uncommon and so having water sprayed over them might be genuinely alarming.

To avoid problems arising, you could:

◆ Arrange for the person to be in the bathroom as the bath is being run and preparations are made, so that they can take in the whole scene as it develops and thus be better prepared.

◆ Try, too, to allow a person some modesty with the use of a strategically placed flannel or loose-fitting underwear, which still allows for washing.

◆ Talk reassuringly as the process is being carried out, especially if a hoist is being used.

When problems do arise, it can all happen suddenly and you have to respond quickly; your aim should be not to make things worse and to find effective ways of calming things down in the least possible time.

Every situation is different, but here are some points to bear in mind:

A younger person might feel nervous and unsettled and might giggle. This should be avoided; the person with dementia will probably take it at face value and interpret it as some kind of mockery, which risks inflaming the situation.

In general try to stay calm in order to avoid the situation escalating. Avoid open questions no matter how appropriate they would normally be. Instead of saying, 'What's wrong?' say something like, 'I can see you are upset.' Say vaguely reassuring things such as, 'Mum, I understand you are unhappy' or 'Ian, we'll get this sorted.' It's a good idea to carry a list of phrases like this in your head if similar situations arise regularly. You should also note any phrases that tend to inflame the situation, which should of course be avoided. All such phrases should be made known to anybody who is regularly involved in the person's care.

Move gradually towards encouraging the person to express their concerns – as and when realistically possible.

Avoid shouted threats or commands. These will almost certainly make the situation worse and should always be avoided despite the understandable exasperation or despair you might well be feeling.

Look for warning signs. A person with dementia can become agitated before an incident actually occurs. Sometimes signs can be spotted, and with the right response it is possible for a difficult situation to be avoided. Something may change in the person's demeanour and there are early signs of agitation. For instance, the person:

◆ Stops making eye contact.
◆ Won't engage in conversation.
◆ Becomes fidgety.
◆ Starts walking around rapidly.

If this happens, here are some things you can do:

◆ Avoid any activity, bathing for instance, that risks causing agitation.

◆ Try to have a change of pace, mood or scene. Make a snack or go out for a walk.

◆ Wait until the signs have passed before engaging in any activities.

Sometimes a person with dementia becomes agitated as a result of hallucinations. They might say they saw a face at the window and express fear that they will be attacked. In general, as with other situations, the best course is to try to get into their reality, and try to talk about what they are experiencing in the hope of defusing the situation.

However, if the person is particularly agitated then you should consider going along with what they are saying – up to a point. Get up, go to the window, have a good look and then come back and say, 'I've had a good look. I can't see anybody there now.' In this way, without actually saying it, you are implying that what they said was true but that you are now able to provide reassurance that everything is all right.

A similar approach could be considered for delusions – unfounded beliefs that, for instance, someone is trying to steal money from them – which is a feature of some types of dementia.

Simply denying their reality won't improve things and risks making the situation worse.

Bear in mind, by the way, that not all hallucinations are unpleasant or threatening – a person might see a colourful bird flying around.

You should aim to deflect the person from their sudden flare-up of emotion. It might seem like a bizarre idea, and it might well be a long shot, but consider leaving the room – if you feel this is safe – and returning a few minutes later wearing a different set of clothes; or, if possible, have someone else come back in your place. Such an unexpected development might just have the effect of taking the wind out of the person's sails, changing the mood and thus allowing you to suggest a cup of tea.

If it proves impossible to pacify a person you should consider, as a last resort, using an argument that you know the person will find persuasive but which is not true.

For example, suppose a man loudly insists at three o' clock in the morning that he must get up and go to work, and that all gentler attempts to dissuade him have failed and the person's behaviour is in danger of creating an unmanageable situation. You tell the person in no uncertain terms that if he does not go back to bed it will be necessary to phone his son (or whoever) and get him to come round to the house, which will involve waking him up in the middle of night and making him late for work the next day.

The point about such strategies is that they will be based on facts within your knowledge. You will know, for example, that the person has always been fond of his son – who is a reasonably powerful character – and that one of the things in life he hates most, which the person knows well, is being late for work. This might just be enough to resolve the situation.

Some people will regard this sort of strategy as morally unacceptable. Although it is based on some truths, the fact is you will not really be intending to make the phone call. There are, however, some situations where the morality of the situation has to be weighed against the need to bring a situation under control. I think strategies like this are acceptable but only as a last resort.

What's more, if they do work they are surely better than the use of powerful drugs.

Ideally, though, they should not be made up on the spur of the moment in response to a crisis but rather thought through in advance, probably as a response to a previous incident.

After an episode has been brought to a conclusion, you should definitely not try to analyse it with the person – who might well have forgotten all about it. It will be far better to reflect on it calmly, perhaps with other people close to the situation, in the hope that lessons can be learned about how best to manage similar situations in the future.

You do need to keep in mind your own safety and develop a knack for assessing when a situation becomes dangerous. If a person larger than you is holding an object that could be a potential weapon, you do have to consider whether to withdraw and contact the authorities.

APPARENTLY INEXPLICABLE BEHAVIOUR

Especially in the later stages, people might do and say things that you simply don't understand. If you keep on asking them questions in an attempt to figure out the meaning, you will probably get nowhere and raise stress levels all round. In these situations you need to practise good communication skills; you also need to be a good detective.

Your starting point should be that there is some logical reason for what is being said or done.

If an elderly man with dementia insists that he needs 'to get the van out and see the men' you could remind him that he is at home, that he can't drive anymore and that there aren't any men anywhere. This would be true but almost certainly unhelpful. You should listen to what is said and repeat back to the person some key words in the hope of engaging with the feelings and concerns the person is experiencing and endeavouring to alleviate them. It is fine to nod vaguely in agreement without actually going along with what is being said.

Later, you should speak to friends and family members in the hope that that they might be able to throw some light on what the person was trying to say. Perhaps, years ago, the man had a job which involved driving to a work site and handing out pay packets to the staff. If you find this out it will be easier, if and when the situation recurs, to engage meaningfully with the man. The message you convey to the person at the time will be that his concerns have been understood.

You should aim to do this without correcting him or bringing him out of his reality.

INAPPROPRIATE BEHAVIOUR

Dementia can lead to people behaving and communicating in uninhibited ways that they would not have done in the past, when they understood the desirability of observing social norms. They might:

◆ Describe a friend or a customer in a restaurant in a derogatory or insulting way, regardless of whether the person can hear them or not.

◆ Swear and make accusations when annoyed about something.

◆ Start talking across another person.

◆ Break wind or pick their nose.

◆ Laugh at things which are serious and not in any way funny.

◆ Make rude or highly critical comments about a person's clothes.

The person might be oblivious to other people's feelings and yet be upset if somebody else did similar things in their presence.

Try to remain calm. Do not draw attention to what the person says or does and move on. If you are in a café or a restaurant it is more difficult. In extreme situations it is probably best to leave; otherwise a discreet word or gesture exchanged with the targeted person might suffice.

One potentially difficult area is sex – one of the most powerful and basic forms of communication there is.

Despite there being much greater openness on the subject of sex in society generally, it remains an area that many people find hard to talk about when it comes to older people with dementia.

On the one hand, in principle, there is no reason why a person with dementia should not continue to enjoy an active sex life with their partner. On the other, dementia can have the effect of changing the ways in which a person approaches sex. Here are some fairly common issues:

◆ A marked increase in sexual desire.

◆ Mechanical and unloving sexual relations; the relief of a
physical desire.

◆ Sex accompanied by a degree of aggression.

◆ Inappropriate sexual approaches – perhaps to a person's
daughter instead of his wife, or a member of staff in a
care home.

*In the case of older people with dementia there can be other
ailments which make satisfactory sexual relations difficult to
achieve – these are matters for a doctor.*

For example, let's say a man with dementia starts to touch a
younger female relative or visitor in a sexual way. She might
instinctively push the man away and say something along the
lines of, 'Get off me, that's disgusting', with a look of revulsion
on her face. However, the message communicated to the man
would be hurtful and upsetting and the chances are that he would
not understand or really learn the message that his behaviour was
inappropriate and unacceptable. Perhaps the woman bore some
resemblance to a girlfriend from the past; perhaps the man was
simply acting in a disinhibited way as a result of his particular
type of dementia.

Here are some guidelines for situations of this kind:

◆ Withdraw calmly so that you are not within touching
distance.

◆ Try if possible to get another person to join you.

◆ Say something which makes it clear who you are: 'Dad, it's Rosie, Mum's upstairs just now.'

◆ Orient him further by telling him, if appropriate, that his wife (i.e. the person with whom sexual contact is appropriate) will be there soon. Perhaps there is a photograph of her that you can point to.

◆ Try to distract the person, change the subject and move on.

◆ Try to give him some object to hold.

Afterwards, discuss the situation with other people involved in the care of the person to consider strategies for dealing with any future incidents.

This is a complex area. A detailed discussion of the subject is beyond the scope of this book. The Alzheimer Society's website contains a great deal of useful information and advice.

PROBLEMATIC WALKING OR 'WANDERING'

The term 'wandering' is far from ideal because it sounds pejorative; it is also very vague – a person might want to walk around for many reasons. Unfortunately nobody seems to have come up with a better word that has caught on. (Some people talk about a person taking little journeys, going sightseeing or going to see what's happening, but these risk being patronizing.) It is a fairly common phenomenon among people with dementia and can cause great concern if it involves the person going outdoors. A related phenomenon is 'pacing', which involves restlessly walking around a lot, though not necessarily going outdoors.

The important point to bear in mind is that the person feels the need to move around for a reason.

It might be a case of boredom, constipation, backache, feeling too hot or a reaction to medication, or perhaps it is as a result of the person having an idea that they have to go and visit someone or report to a place of work from long ago. Perhaps the person led a very active physical life in which case it would be a good idea to lay on as much exercise as possible, which might reduce their desire to move about at other times.

A bit of detective work can help to throw light on the reasons why they are doing this, which in turn might enable you to encourage the person to communicate their feelings and concerns to possibly provide some relief.

However, you do also need to be aware of safety issues. Here are some ways of addressing the phenomenon:

◆ You can of course lock all doors to the outside. There is clearly an argument in favour of doing this at night – you might well do it anyway; during the day this might seem drastic. If you lock doors, the danger is that you make people feel restricted and restless, and also reduce their opportunities for taking exercise.

◆ You could install discreet alarms on external doors.

◆ If there is a garden, consider leaving the house doors unlocked whilst ensuring that the garden is secure.

◆ Mirrors and hanging beads on the backs of external doors have been found to discourage people from trying to open them. These objects appear to send a message that there is some obstacle to opening the door – though they are not of course foolproof.

◆ Use masking tape to create a grid pattern in front of the door, similar to a box junction on a road.

◆ External glass doors through which sunlight streams can be an attractive draw and might encourage a person to head outside. Consider installing curtains or placing pieces of furniture in front of such doors on sunny days.

◆ Cover door handles with squares of materials or curtains.

◆ If a person seems very keen to go outside it might be a good idea simply to put a coat on and accompany them. Try to engage them in conversation to get an idea of what is on their mind, and after a while gently steer them back towards home with the promise of a cup of tea.

If a person does go missing, the situation is urgent and the police are usually contacted. At least one police force in England has now provided some people known to be vulnerable, including some with dementia, with wearable GPS tracking devices on the basis that this is quicker, not to mention cheaper, than sending out police cars or even helicopters to look for them. While there are clear advantages to this, there are those who think it wrong to tag a person with dementia in the same way as some convicted criminals.

'SUNDOWNING'

This expression refers to a series of behaviours which sometimes occur in the late afternoon/early evening, such as:

◆ Increased disorientation.
◆ Reduced mental processing powers.
◆ Agitation.
◆ Confusion.

There are various theories as to why this happens, for example blood sugar level issues or out-of-sync daily rhythms. By no means will every person with dementia experience this phenomenon. If it does happen, you firstly need to accept that communication might be more difficult and that this will not be a good time to engage in activities or outings. Probably the simplest and most appropriate response is to create a calm atmosphere, be with the person and perhaps take them for a gentle stroll or give them a relaxing bath or massage.

PEOPLE WHOSE FIRST LANGUAGE IS NOT ENGLISH

There is a particular situation that can arise as dementia progresses, whereby a person who came to the UK years ago, and then learned English, starts to lose some or all of what they learned and reverts to their mother tongue. By the time this happens the person may be living in a mainly English-speaking environment and their loss of English will be problematic.

The person will not be able to re-learn English – nor should they be expected to since this will involve a lot of brain work. It might be necessary, if possible, to adapt the person's life to reintroducing the language they feel comfortable with. Perhaps their language will become a combination of their mother tongue and English. Family members might be able to help with interpretation and make a list of key words from the mother tongue that the person uses regularly and which those helping to look after them could become familiar with.

11

Wills, Powers of Attorney, Living Wills and Personal Wishes

We are generally encouraged by lawyers and others to make wills. It is good advice: wills should enable people to avoid arguments over money and property after their deaths. In the last forty years or so the whole subject of the expression of people's wishes in legal documents has broadened out to include other important areas, such as issues relating to health and welfare when a person becomes incapacitated.

All such documents constitute a very important area of communication since they set out some of the most fundamental wishes a person can express – matters of life and death and the destination of their estate.

These issues are all complicated by the onset of dementia, which will result in a gradual loss of capacity to make decisions and express wishes. The net result is that whereas a person with mental capacity is able to communicate their testamentary and other wishes until very near the time of their death, a person with dementia is unable to do this.

WILLS

If a person made a will before the onset of dementia, you should check that the document still reflects their wishes regarding their estate, legacies and issues such as burial versus cremation. In addition, there might be grandchildren or other close relatives who have come along since the document was originally prepared to whom the person would like to leave something. If any changes are to be made you should enlist the assistance of a solicitor and discuss the person's condition with them. The solicitor will want to be satisfied that the person fully understands the nature of any changes to be made.

If the person with dementia has never made a will, you should give serious consideration to encouraging them to do so now.

POWER OF ATTORNEY

A power of attorney is appropriate when you want to have the authority of the person to carry out certain specific functions on their behalf. It can only be validly signed by the person if they retain sufficient mental capacity. In the early stages this should not present a problem, so long as it is clear they understand the nature and purpose of the document and are happy to sign it. If you are in doubt about their capacity, a professional, such as a doctor, solicitor or speech and language therapist, should be consulted for appropriate advice and assistance.

A common scenario is that a person with dementia finds it increasingly difficult to keep a track on household bills and generally manage their own financial affairs. In England and Wales there is a document called a Lasting Power of Attorney, which comes in two parts – firstly, property and financial, and then health and welfare. The property and financial part allows the attorney, or attorneys, to deal with all matters including the sale of property – *before and after a person loses mental capacity.*

Unfortunately, the person will realize that the granting of a power of attorney is more evidence of their failing mental powers. Therefore the matter should be handled sensitively with much emphasis placed on the advantages to all concerned. When checking and paying bills, the attorney should act discreetly, preferably in such a way that the person is not aware that it is happening. In time, the person will gradually become less and less aware of such matters.

You should ensure, however, that for as long as makes sense, the person does have some money in their pocket or purse to spend at local shops, on outings or small gifts. In this way they can continue to enjoy a degree of financial independence and express the natural desire to be generous.

LIVING WILLS

In recent years there has been a significant public demand in many countries for an answer to the question: 'How can I make sure my wishes regarding my welfare, medical treatment and interventions are communicated and respected if I become incapacitated?'

The answer in many countries is living wills. They originated in America in the late 1960s and are now widely available in many countries. They aim to enable a person, when still capable of understanding and dealing with their own affairs, to grant authority to named people to make decisions that reflect their wishes when they become mentally incapacitated.

Examples of subjects covered in living wills include:

◆ Admission to a care home.

◆ Whether a person should be fed via tubes.

◆ Whether a person should be resuscitated in the event of, say, heart failure.

◆ Pain relief.

In the absence of any form of living will, decisions will be taken by relatives and doctors. In the past, with regard to medical matters, the doctors would have said to relatives, 'Here are the facts, here are the choices, what do *you* want us to do?' Nowadays things have changed; the doctors say, 'Here are the facts, here are the choices, what would *the person* have wanted us to do?' This might result in appropriate decisions being taken, but there can be uncertainty and agonizing over what to do and who exactly makes the decisions.

With an appropriate legal document, named people, usually trusted relatives or friends, have the authority to take decisions they are reasonably confident reflect the person's wishes.

These documents, which have had various names in different places over the years – advance health-care directives, personal directives, advance decisions – are clearly relevant and appropriate for people with dementia. In England and Wales, the health and welfare element of Lasting Powers of Attorney gives named relatives the right to seek to carry out the wishes of the person when they lose mental capacity. The documents give the attorney a wide range of powers and it is also possible to add in other specific wishes the person wants to have mentioned.

Such legal documents can be downloaded at *gov.uk/power-of-attorney*, though they can only be used after you have registered them with the Office of the Public Guardian, which at the time of writing costs £110 per document.

Similar documents are available in Scotland and Northern Ireland.

Here are a number of general points to bear in mind.

Whatever type of document you think is appropriate, don't put it off. If you wait until the person has become mentally incapacitated it will not be possible to have documents signed and it might be necessary to go through the courts to get authority to look after the person's affairs.

Living wills can help to relieve the burden on you and other people involved in the care of the person if and when decisions about life-saving treatment need to be made.

Any document can only be an expression of wishes at one point in time. Accordingly, you might want to consider updates now and then if the person has the capacity to do this.

The fact that a person has signed a living will or similar document is not a guarantee. It does not mean it will be possible to carry out all of their wishes to the letter.

The person should be discouraged from including impractical conditions. For example, that they only want a particular doctor to treat them or that no treatment should be administered during the night.

Timing. One of your challenges will be to raise the topic with the person at a time when they know they have a problem but before they lose mental capacity. You will have to be diplomatic and sensitive.

Is it what the person wants? It is important too that you ascertain whether the person really wants to go through the process of obtaining and signing a living will or any other document. The fact is there are plenty of people who simply trust their nearest and dearest to do the right thing.

This whole area involves fairly complex legal issues. Therefore, if you think a will or some form of power of attorney might be right for the person in your life, it is vital that you take action and seek appropriate professional advice sooner rather than later.

INFORMAL WISHES

Communicating wishes about things that will happen around the time of a person's death is not just about legal formalities and life and death issues.

Towards the end of their lives many people talk to their close relatives and friends about a whole range of things they would like to happen as they approach this time. Some are of great personal significance; others could be seen as more whimsical or sentimental. Relatives and very close friends make mental notes, discuss issues, build up a picture of the person's wishes and then do their best to make sure they are respected.

Dementia in the later stages can rob people of this form of communication and as a result many topics will simply be subject to guesswork when the time comes.

Accordingly, I think there is a strong argument in favour of picking up on any comments a person makes before they start to lose the ability to engage in conversations of this type and to really find out what their wishes are. It will be a communicative challenge to find ways to discuss these things with a person without upsetting them too much. Make a note of the points and do your best to see that at least some are honoured.

Informal wishes of this kind will not be legally binding nor would they involve significant amounts of money or life and death issues – those things should be dealt with in wills, powers of attorney and living wills.

Here are some examples:

◆ Small gifts of personal items to particular people.
◆ Attitude to going into a care home.
◆ Thoughts on being looked after at home.
◆ Preferred people to be with in the last stages of life.
◆ Choice of music to play in the last stages of life and also at the funeral.
◆ Who should speak or sing or recite poetry at the funeral.
◆ Notice in newspapers.
◆ Words on gravestone.
◆ Who might write an obituary.

◆ Organization of memorial event/planting tree, etc.
◆ Scattering of ashes.

This sort of thing will not be for everybody; some families would just find it too awkward or painful. As with other similar issues, there are a lot people with dementia who will be content to trust their loved ones to take appropriate decisions.

Nevertheless, there is surely something to be said for enabling a person to communicate wishes which you will then carry out. On a more selfish note, you will help to reduce the amount of guesswork you have to undertake when it comes to funeral and other related arrangements.

12

Care Homes

This chapter is about situations where a decision is taken, or circumstances arise, which result in a person with dementia moving away from their familiar home environment. One main reason is when the person goes into residential care – this could be a permanent move or for a set period of respite care.

Major events like this involve a lot of transitional change, which will almost certainly be unsettling and stressful for a person with dementia.

HELPING TO MAKE THE TRANSITION

For the actual period when a major transition in a person's life takes place, you should try to set aside some time so that you – and other family members or close friends – are available for as much time as possible before, during and for a time after the move takes place, so that you can be on hand to provide reassurance and respond to any problems that arise.

It can be hard for people with dementia to answer questions that might be put to them by members of staff. You or another trusted person will doubtless be there some of the time and will act as their advocate. Staff will want to have relevant information about the person and there will be forms to complete. However, they might not cover some points you regard as most important; so in addition to completing any form provided by the care home, you should provide a simple document – a personal factsheet – providing staff with the things they need to know in order to make the person's experience as smooth as possible.

Some writers refer to a document of this kind as a passport or a profile.

You should aim to let staff know as much as possible about the person in the fewest possible words. You know that this person has had a life and you want to make staff feel the same way. Ideally it should not exceed one A4 piece of paper. If it is longer it is more likely not to be read and absorbed by busy staff.

You will doubtless talk to a member of staff when you arrive at the care home and have an opportunity to explain important points of particular relevance – but there will be lots of other members of staff involved, hence the importance of providing a simple document to be placed with the person's notes. You should seek assurance that all members of staff coming into contact with the person will familiarize themselves with the information you provide.

In addition you should speak to staff members whenever you visit, tell them more about the person and answer any questions they might have.

You could probably write screeds about the person you know so well, but you need to adopt a practical and realistic attitude. Staff are busy and have lots of people to care for. Accordingly, you should whittle down what you want to say to some vital points that get over what you most want the staff to know. It is probably best that factsheets are not seen by the person with dementia.

Here are some examples of the sort of information to include; there might be some duplication with the forms you are asked to complete by the home but the fact that important points are repeated does not matter:

What is the person normally called? If the person's name is Ronald but he is invariably called Ronnie or Ron, then calling him Ronald will probably cause confusion. He will understand that someone is trying to talk to him from their eye contact and other bits of non-verbal communication but will have difficulty working out why he is not being called by the name he is familiar with.

Some staff assume that everybody likes to addressed by their first name and this is certainly the norm – however, this might not always be the case and the person's preference should be made clear.

Words the person uses for everyday things. For instance, if the person always refers to a cup of tea as a 'brew' or a 'cup of char', mention this. Similarly, if the person always talks of 'spending a penny', then put it down.

Subjects to avoid. If a person was greatly upset by, for example, the recent death of a spouse, clearly staff should be advised to steer clear of this.

Any particularly strong food and drink likes and dislikes?

Shaving foam or gel?

Whether keen on spending some time out of doors whenever possible.

Details of people who are likely to visit regularly. In this way the staff will not have to quiz the person when a visitor arrives at the home. Including photographs will make things even smoother.

Any particular eccentricities? If a person likes to wear a particular hat even though it might be unnecessary in a warm home this should be mentioned.

A few phrases that go the heart of who the person is. 'He was always a hard worker.' 'She never could stand political correctness.' Such phrases will help to bring the person to life for staff.

When the person prefers to get up in the morning.

Does the person like group activities? Or do they prefer to do things one to one?

In care homes a person will have regular reviews that will consider all aspects of their care and general well-being. Once more, these are meetings where you should act as the person's advocate. It will be advisable to make preparations for such review meetings by speaking to the person in advance to hear about any concerns or comments.

Of course, none of this precludes the person from speaking up about any concerns they might have, too.

In addition, some of the headline historical facts of the person's life should be included. Here are some examples:

◆ City or town raised in.

◆ Schooling.

◆ Work – main area of skill.

◆ Interests and hobbies – it would probably be a good idea to mention a few favourite films or books or holiday destinations, which could provide material for some chit-chat.

◆ Religious beliefs and practices – if an important part of the person's life.

The hope and expectation is that the staff will soon develop their own relationships with the person. Staff should then see relatives and friends as a resource to be consulted from time to time for more information and answers to queries that might arise. There can be a high turnover of staff in care homes and so taking the initiative to talk to them and ensure they are familiar with the factsheet will always be desirable.

What you want to avoid is the recognized phenomenon of a member of staff attending the funeral of a former resident and discovering things about them they didn't know and which, had they known them sooner, might have enhanced the quality of care provided.

The person's room

It is a good idea to have something on the person's door which they recognize as relating to them. Photographs are often used but they can be confusing. A woman with advanced dementia might look at a recent picture of herself and think it is her mother. Trial and error is the key – perhaps an old poster, a picture of a favourite pet or an item of clothing. Apart from contributing to a sense of identity, the right item will help to prevent the person from going into the wrong room.

A person's room should have a number of carefully selected personal objects – familiar items of furniture, photographs, holiday souvenirs, pictures, books, a rummage box perhaps – things which are all about continuity.

Make sure the person has a plentiful supply of clothes. There is nothing worse than seeing people wearing other people's clothes, which look wrong and, worse still, don't fit properly.

Nowadays some rooms in care homes are unfurnished and this gives maximum scope for personalization with furniture as well as smaller items. Furniture should not be placed in such a way as to block pictures or other items on the walls, which should be placed at the right height for the person to be able to see them clearly.

If possible try to ensure that the person with dementia can still be a host – something they have probably enjoyed doing for a large part of their lives – in however small a way. This might just be a case of having a kettle with tea and coffee and some biscuits in their room.

Day care

People with dementia will quite often attend day care on a regular basis. A brief factsheet containing certain key bits of information for the staff will almost certainly help to smooth over any potential communication difficulties in this situation, too.

Hospital

From time to time it might be necessary for a person with dementia to go into hospital for treatment. Transitions to and from hospital with their busy and noisy environments can be particularly stressful and alarming for people with dementia. Bear in mind, too, that by no means all staff will have had dementia-awareness training – though nowadays more information about the person will be sought on admission than would have been the case in the past. However, as with care homes, you should provide staff with a few points you think are most important in a brief factsheet. Perhaps a copy could be left in the person's bedside cabinet.

Another point about hospitals is that relatives and friends might find that they are only allowed to visit at fixed times. This is in contrast to children's wards where it has been realized in many cases that the presence of relatives and friends at any time of day or night can help to make the hospital stay easier and less stressful for all concerned. It should be the same with people with dementia. The presence of somebody close can reduce anxiety and might result in shorter hospital stays.

Not only that but it means somebody can be on hand to answer questions from staff and be an advocate for the person when it

comes to any matters that are causing concern. If this means
a relative bedding down on a chair next to the person's bed
then in my view this should be permitted unless operationally
impracticable – however this is something you might have to
fight for.

If a person is in hospital and able to move around, you might
consider giving them a small postcard-sized document with some
basic information such as their name and which ward they are in.
This could be worn on a cord around the neck or on a wristband
– somewhere obvious. Similarly, a plastic folder containing an
information sheet could be attached to a Zimmer frame. Another
possibility would be a bag that goes round the waist.

Moving in with relatives

A person with dementia might move in with relatives or friends
on a temporary or permanent basis. It might also happen that
a person has a full-time live-in carer. In either case, the person
should have or retain areas of the house that contain a lot of
familiar things so that they have the best chance of adjusting to
the new arrangement as quickly as possible.

In Conclusion

I really hope that you have found some things of use in this book. Looking after a person with dementia can be very hard at times; the nature of the condition, especially in the later stages, can stretch anyone to the limits of endurance on occasion. This is a fact that should be acknowledged. However, there can be great rewards too, and the best possible communication makes them more achievable.

Communication is a major subject; it goes to the heart of what it is to be human. The more we can do to keep the channels open and functioning as well as possible for as long as possible, the better we will make life for people with dementia. In the process we can help to reduce the high degree of stress which can undoubtedly be associated with the condition at times. It might also be the case that the person will be able to continue to enjoy a greater degree of independence and stay in their own home for a bit longer.

Although there is a great deal that can be said on the subject of communication and people with dementia, I believe there are a few underlying general principles which go to the heart of the matter and which you should always try to keep at the forefront of your mind:

The person can't change, so you have to.

The old ways of communicating won't work any more.

Minimize the load placed on a person's mental-processing powers.

Keep any new learning to an absolute minimum.

Avoid direct questions where possible. Tell, don't ask.

Don't correct or contradict.

Sources and Acknowledgements

In order to write this book, I drew on a number of sources both formal and informal.

In the first place there was my experience of working as a speech and language therapist during which I encountered a wide variety of people and situations. I was struck by the communication difficulties relatives, friends and carers often experienced, and their feelings that not much could be done to make things better. It was at this time, as I looked for ways of trying to explain effective techniques, that the idea of a straightforward, non-academic handbook came to me.

I follow the news on television, radio and also, increasingly, via the internet. The large number of features related to dementia provides striking evidence of just how many people's lives are affected by the condition. New reports appear virtually on a daily basis: abusive behaviour in care homes, medical breakthroughs, recommended lifestyle changes, alterations to accommodation that make life easier, personal accounts of carers, and much else besides. They have provided valuable information, new perspectives and new lines of enquiry about the kinds of problems and issues people with dementia and those caring for them experience all the time; and in most cases communication issues are highly relevant.

I read and considered a diverse range of books, articles and leaflets. If you are involved in the care of a person with dementia I would encourage you to read about the subject. A good place to start is the large number of helpful pamphlets issued by local health authorities and organizations such as the Alzheimer's Society and BUPA. These pamphlets are generally available online; paper copies will also be available from the organizations themselves, health centres, social service offices and libraries.

I am particularly grateful to Professor Mary Marshall, an emeritus professor at the University of Stirling and director of the Dementia Services Development Centre until 2005. She is a leading expert on many aspects of dementia care and has served on numerous boards and committees working with older people, including the Royal Commission on Long Term Care of the Elderly. Professor Marshall kindly read the manuscript and made many wise comments, criticisms and suggestions, the great majority of which have been incorporated into the book.

I am also grateful to Eileen Richardson, the Library & Information Service Manager at the Dementia Services Development Centre in the Iris Murdoch Building at the University of Stirling who assisted greatly with locating books and articles.

Nikki Read and Giles Lewis, my editors at Constable & Robertson, provided valuable help and guidance along the way. My thanks also to Nicky Gyopari for her expert checking and correction of the text.

There are a number of people in my extended family who have been living with dementia for a considerable length of time. My involvement with and observation of the challenges faced by them and their closest relatives has been educational.

Writing a book is a journey. I am fortunate that I did not have to go through it alone. Judy was, as always, by my side.

Useful Websites

The following list contains a small selection of websites which contain useful information. There are many more and I would encourage you to carry out searches of relevance to your own particular situation – there is a great deal of help and information available.

Please note that although some of the main websites have 'Alzheimer's' in their titles they are concerned with dementia of all types.

Alzheimer's Society
www.alzheimers.org.uk
Note the Alzheimer's Society covers England, Wales and Northern Ireland.

Alzheimer Scotland – Action on Dementia
www.alzscot.org

NHS
www.nhs.uk/conditions/dementia-guide/pages/about-dementia.aspx

Dementia Services Development Centre
www.dementia.stir.ac.uk

Bupa
www.bupa.co.uk/health-information/Directory/D/dementia

Action on Hearing Loss
www.actiononhearingloss.org.uk

Royal National Institute of Blind People
www.rnib.org.uk

YouTube
www.youtube.com

The National Archives
www.nationalarchives.gov.uk/films

Scottish Screen Archive
www.ssa.nls.uk

Share-Time Pictures
www.sharetimepictures.com.au/Judi-Parkinson---Producer.php

Memory Bank
www.memory-bank.org

Nordoff Robbins
www.nordoff-robbins.org.uk

Active Minds
www.active-minds.co.uk

Talking Mats
www.talkingmats.com

Bibliography

BOOKS

Aldridge, D. (ed) (2000) *Music Therapy in Dementia Care. More New Voices.* London: Jessica Kingsley.

Bayley, J. (1999) *Iris: A Memoir of Iris Murdoch.* London: Abacus.

Bell, V. and Troxel, D. (2002) *The Best Friends Approach to Alzheimer's Care.* Baltimore: Health Professions Press.

Bonner, C. (2005) *Reducing Stress-Related Behaviours in People with Dementia. Care-based Therapy.* London: Jessica Kingsley.

Bourgeois, M. S. (2007) *Memory Books and other Graphic Cuing Systems: Practical Communication and Memory Aids for Adults with Dementia.* Baltimore, MD: Health Professions Press.

Buijsen, H. (2005) *The Simplicity of Dementia: A Guide for Family and Carers.* London: Jessica Kingsley.

Cheston, R. and Bender, M. (2003) *Understanding Dementia: The Man with the Worried Eyes.* London: Jessica Kingsley.

De Klerk-Rubin, V. (2006) *Validation Techniques for Dementia Care: The Family Guide to Improving Communication.* Baltimore: Health Professions Press.

Downs, M. and Bowers, B. (eds) (2008) *Excellence in Dementia Care. Research into Practice.* Maidenhead: Open University Press

Fournier, E. (2007) *J'ai Commencé mon Eternité. Survivre au Déclin de l'Autre.* Quebec: Les Editions de l'Homme.

Fournier, E. (2008) *La Mère d'Edith. L'Alzheimer en trait d'union.* Quebec: Les Editions de l'Homme.

Giuliano, B. (1996) *Dementia Does Hurt.* Narellan, NSW: Rose Education.

Grealy, J., McMullen, H. and Grealy, J. (2005) *Dementia Care: A Practical Photographic Guide.* Oxford: Blackwell Publishing.

Hodgson, H. (1995) *Alzheimer's: Finding the Words: A Communication Guide for those who Care.* Minneapolis, MN: Chronimed Publishing.

Jones, G. M. M. and Miesen, B. M. L. (2004) *Caregiving in Dementia: Research and Applications Vol 3.* Hove, UK and New York, NY: Brunner-Routledge Taylor and Francis Group.

Killick, J. and Allan, K. (2001) *Communication and the Care of People with Dementia.* Buckingham: Open University Press.

Killick, J. and Craig, C. (2012) *Creativity and Communication in Persons with Dementia.* London: Jessica Kingsley.

Kitwood, T. (1997) *Dementia Reconsidered. The Person Comes First.* Buckingham: Open University Press.

Kuhn, D. and Verity, J. (2008) *The Art of Dementia Care.* New York, NY: Thomson Delmar Learning.

Magnusson, S. (2014) *Where Memories Go.* London: Two Roads.

Powell, J. (2000). *Care to Communicate: Helping the Older Person with Dementia.* London: Hawker Publications.

Rau, M.T. (1993) *Coping with Communication Challenges in Alzheimer's Disease.* San Diego, California: Singular Publishing Group.

Sanderson, H. and Bailey, G. (2014) *Personalisation and Dementia: A Guide for Person Centred Practice.* London: Jessica Kingsley.

Santo Pietro, M. J. and Ostuni, E. (1997) *Successful Communication with Alzheimer's Disease Patients. An In-Service Manual.* Oxford: Butterworth-Heinemann.

Suchet, J. (2011) *My Bonnie: How Dementia Stole the Love of My Life.* London: Harper.

Tappen, R. M. (1997) *Interventions for Alzheimer's Disease: A Caregiver's Complete Reference*. Baltimore, MD: Health Professions Press.

Whitman, L. (ed) (2009) *Telling Tales about Dementia. Experiences of Caring*. London: Jessica Kingsley.

Young, T., Manthorp, C. and Howells, D. (2010) *Communication and Dementia: New Perspectives, New Approaches*. Madrid: Editorial Aresta.

ARTICLES

Baum, C. and Edwards, D. F. (2003) 'What a Person with Alzheimer's Disease can do: a Tool for Communication about Everyday Activities' in *Alzheimer's Care Quarterly*, 4 (2): 108–18.

Cox, S., Murphy, J. and Gray, C. (2008) 'How Effective is the Talking Mats Approach?' in *The Journal of Dementia Care*, 16 (3): 35–8.

Elkins, Z. (2011) 'Communication Bridges for Patients with Dementia' in *Primary Health Care*, 21 (10): 16–19.

Ellis, J. (2003) 'Music and Communication in a Person with Advanced Alzheimer's Disease' in *Signpost*, 8 (1): 27–9.

Ellis, M. and Astell, A. (2011) 'Adaptive Interaction: a New Approach to Communication' in *The Journal of Dementia Care*, 19(3): 24–6.

Gill, A. A. (2007) 'Father' in In *Previous Convictions. Assignments from Here and There* (London: Phoenix), 16–21.

Gleeson, M. and Timmins, F. (2004) 'Touch: a Fundamental Aspect of Communication with Older People Experiencing Dementia' in *Nursing Older People*, 16 (2): 18–21.

Goldfein, S. (2007) 'Supporting People with Early Stage Alzheimer's Disease: Communication Considerations' in *Alzheimer's Care Quarterly*, 8 (1): 26–33.

Haak, N. J. (2006) 'Communication the Heart of Caregiving' in *Alzheimer's Care Quarterly*, 7 (2): 77–83.

Hobbs, L. (2009) 'Communication and Dementia: How Can We Help Families?' in *The Journal of Dementia Care*, 17 (2): 20–1.

obson, P. (2012) 'Communication. Making Sense of What People with Dementia Say' in *British Journal of Healthcare Assistants*, 6 (7): 334–7.

Jootun, D. and McGhee, G. (2011) 'Effective Communication with People who have Dementia' in *Nursing Standard*, 25 (25): 40–6.

Murphy, J., Gray, C. M. and Cox, Sylvia. (2007) *Communication and Dementia. How Talking Mats can help People with Dementia to Express Themselves.* Project Report: Joseph Rowntree Foundation.

Parkinson, J. (2010) 'The Creation of Non-Verbal Communication Tools to Assist Social Interactions for People with Dementia and Alzheimer's Disease' in *Signpost*, 15 (1): 33–7.

Ryan, E. B., Bannister, K. A. and Anas, A. P. (2009) 'The Dementia Narrative: Writing to Reclaim Social Identity' in *Journal of Aging Studies*, 23 (3): 145–57.

Stevenson, L. (2008) *Hearing the Voice: Improving Communication with a Person with Dementia.* Study Guide: Dementia Services Development Centre, Stirling University.

Schweitzer, P. and Bruce, E. (2008) 'Reminiscence, Communication and Conversation' in *The Journal of Dementia Care*, 16(5): 18–20.

Walker, B. (2007) 'Communication: Building up a Toolkit of Helpful Responses' in *The Journal of Dementia Care*, 15 (1): 28–30.

Index